Being an E-learner in Health and Social Care

E-learni
health a
stages. I
whether
    Being
and thei
being an
provides
learning
teaching
discusse

- skill
- the
- clini
- asse

Being a
students
in nursir

Julie San
Social C:

Liz Smit
Social C:

Being an E-learner in Health and Social Care

A student's guide

Julie Santy and Liz Smith

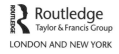

Routledge
Taylor & Francis Group

LONDON AND NEW YORK

First published 2007 by Routledge
2 Park Square, Milton Park, Abingdon, Oxon, OX14 4RN

Simultaneously published in the USA and Canada
by Routledge
270 Madison Avenue, New York, NY 10016

Routledge is an imprint of the Taylor & Francis Group, an informa business

© 2007 Julie Santy and Liz Smith

Typeset in Sabon by Florence Production Ltd, Stoodleigh, Devon
Printed and bound in Great Britain by TJ International Ltd,
Padstow, Cornwall

British Library Cataloguing in Publication Data
A catalogue record for this book is available from the British Library

Library of Congress Cataloging in Publication Data
A catalog record for this book has been requested.

ISBN10: 0–415–40141–0 (hbk)
ISBN10: 0–415–40142–9 (pbk)
ISBN10: 0–203–96175–7 (ebk)

ISBN13: 978–0–415–40141–8 (hbk)
ISBN13: 978–0–415–40142–5 (pbk)
ISBN13: 978–0–203–96175–9 (ebk)

Contents

Illustrations

Figures

Tables

Introduction

Many programmes and courses in health and social care practice now incorporate aspects of electronic learning (e-learning) to support study. This mode of learning is new, interesting, rewarding, exciting and effective. However, for those students embarking on e-learning for the first time it can also be, to some degree, daunting and anxiety provoking, depending, of course, on the student's own circumstances and previous experiences. The novelty of this method of learning is also a challenge for tutors and lecturers using e-learning for the first time.

You may be a qualified or beginner health or social care professional or a teacher working with students of health and social care. The aim of this guide is to help students and tutors for whom e-learning is a relatively new experience to understand what is expected of them in this new situation, and to get to grips with the learning methods, technology and terminology. It will also act as a reference text once your e-learning experience is underway. All you need to get going with e-learning is access to the Internet and some enthusiasm for learning – and maybe a little help and support! You don't need to be a whiz with computers, just to have a desire to learn.

The guide will assume no previous knowledge of e-learning or computer and technical terminology, and it will explain how e-learning works, how to make a start with the technology, what its advantages are, the role of the student and the role of the tutor. It will also help you to prepare yourself for e-learning by encouraging you to think about the issues that may hinder or enhance your learning in this new situation.

Being an e-learner *can* be fun and very rewarding and it will enhance your practice with patients and clients. Being an e-tutor is equally stimulating. You may find that you don't want to go back to more traditional approaches in the future! It can, however, be quite daunting if you are learning to be an e-learner at the same time as trying to learn about the content of your course and module. If we could give you only three pieces of advice they would be these:

- Seek help from your tutor right from day one – that's what the tutor is there for and they would rather you let them know when you need help or support than find out that you are struggling when it is too late.

- Set time aside for e-learning – it's certainly a flexible approach to learning but it can't be done in five minutes here and there. The biggest mistake students make is to assume that their learning can just 'fit in' around everything else in their lives.
- Make the most of the learning community with your fellow students – get to know them and make an effort to allow them to get to know you. Socialization in learning is vital and you will enjoy it so much more if you get into the thick of it!

This book is based on our experiences of working with health and social care students online. Although we have some experience of this, we do not consider ourselves to be 'technical' experts, nor do we think we need to be. We feel that we can offer you practical advice about how to make the best of e-learning opportunities, even if you perceive yourself to be very much a novice technically. The reason we can do this is because we understand how it feels to be technically challenged.

How to use this book

This book has been designed with the student who is new to e-learning in mind. For this reason we have tried to use as little jargon as possible. We have also, however, recognized the need for you to know the meaning of some of the common terms used in everyday e-learning. We have highlighted new terms in bold in the text and have provided explanations of these in the Glossary at the end of the book so that you can look them up if you need to. We also highlight a large number of websites and web pages useful to students and professionals in health and social care. In order to make these easier to access, we have included a list of websites and their addresses or **URLs** in the Appendix.

You may, however, be a more experienced e-learning student who wants to understand the issues in a bit more detail. You might also be an e-learning tutor who wants to think about the issues that directly affect your own students. We, therefore, expect that you will use this book in a variety of ways:

- As a reader – to be worked through chapter by chapter before or during the early stages of an e-learning experience.
- As a tutor to help with ideas about delivering e-learning to a range of different students and in different ways.
- As a 'cook book' to dip in to when issues arise during your e-learning experience – in which case you may wish to use the index at the end of the book to identify where you can find the material you need.
- As a more experienced e-learner to check up on issues arising from researching possible online courses you may wish to undertake.

You will find a number of activities and examples within the text. These are designed to help you to think about how the issues raised in the book apply specifically to you and to help you to make sense of how e-learning can work for you. Although they may seem to be specific to some areas of practice, they are designed to help all health and social care practitioners understand the e-learning process. We have tried to use a wide variety of examples.

Setting some time aside to look at the examples and undertake the activities will help in informing your learning and we recommend that you do as many as you can over the period of your development as an e-learner.

Our experience has shown that many learners and their teachers find learning and teaching online a liberating and enjoyable experience. We hope that you will use this book to help you to get the e-learning bug.

1 E-learning in health and social care

Introduction

The aim of this chapter is to give you an overview of the development, meaning and value of **e-learning** in health and social care. This will help you to think about where e-learning has come from and what its value, as a way of learning, is likely to be for you. It will also help you to identify the pitfalls you are likely to face as an e-learner. The chapter will focus on the current education culture in health and social care education as this is the context in which you will be learning. It will also provide you with an understanding of the background to some of the specific issues around e-learning in health and social care. This will include a discussion of the advantages of e-learning for you and your colleagues and help you to develop a positive attitude towards the process.

What is e-learning?

In order to explain the meaning and value of e-learning, we must begin with the **Internet** – commonly known as the **World Wide Web (Web or www)**. The arrival of the Internet has been the main catalyst for the fact that digital technology is changing how we do business and live our lives. With a worldwide population of around 6.5 billion, one Internet usage survey (ComScore 2006) claims that there are as many as 694 million people using the Internet (as of May 2006). It is important to remember that, although this represents a large percentage of the world's population, there are large tracts of developing countries that have little or no Internet access at all. You could argue that such poor and isolated communities need the education that **online** access promises even more than wealthy communities. It is also worth remembering that poorer communities in wealthier countries have relatively low access and usage of the Internet generally.

The Internet is an ever expanding electronic **network** of computers that operates worldwide, providing access to millions of resources. It enables each computer to have an address that is accessible to all other Internet-connected computers. It has actually been around in some form since the early 1960s, but its use burgeoned during the 1990s, so much so that it has become an integral part of everyday life for the many people across the globe who use it to access information, work, play and to communicate with others.

Radio-based systems now allow transmission of information without a physical connection. The advent of **wireless** communication means that Internet users can take a computer away from the traditional desk and use it remotely anywhere a radio signal is available. Many of these computers are now very small – not much bigger than a mobile telephone or a small book. We can see people using the Internet in hotel foyers, coffee shops and railway stations, as well as in their homes, schools, colleges and universities. Yet, if someone had said, even perhaps only in the early 1990s, that all this would be possible today they would have been accused of being somewhat crazy. There is a saying that every person on the globe is now only six or seven connections away from any other.

It is important to stress again, however, that access to the Internet is not universal. Those people who are disengaged from society, socially excluded, living in poverty or in remote parts of the world, for example, are as yet unable to engage in this new approach to many aspects of life. One could argue that it is now the responsibility of better off governments and individuals across the globe to ensure that such communities and individuals are enabled to connect to the Internet in order to ensure that the gap between those who have and those who have not does not become wider. As a health and social care professional this is something of which you should be very much aware.

Internet technology is also starting to have an impact on the way that we deliver health and social care. Not only does it provide access to information about patients and clients, but also it allows developments in care such as 'telemedicine'. This is where technology, including audio and video, is used for medical diagnosis and patient care when the health care practitioner and client are at a distance, such as in remote areas of countries like Scotland and Australia. Many support groups for people with distressing medical conditions or specific social problems are often now conducted using the Internet (see Box 1.1).

The availability of the Internet has large potential advantages for learning across all age groups. Most schools, and almost every university and college across the globe, now have high-speed Internet access. Teachers increasingly use **information and communications technology (ICT)** to bring their teaching to life (Department for Education and Skills (DfES) 2005). E-learning is a term that you may have heard many times, yet you might still be uncertain of its real meaning and relevance to you. It is a concept that is often referred to in relation to health and social care education and practice. It is important that, before you set out on your e-learning journey, you understand where e-learning has come from and what relevance it has to your education and practice and that of your colleagues.

E-learning has a number of related terms that, essentially, mean the same thing. The most common ones are:

Box 1.1

An example of online patient/client support online: the Tuberculosis Survival Project

http://www.tbsurvivalproject.org (accessed 24 August 2006)

This website was created in recognition of the fact that the emotional and psychological support that many patients with TB or multi-drug-resistant tuberculosis (MDR-TB) receive is inadequate. Being treated and cured of TB/MDR-TB is not just about taking medication. There are many factors that can lead to treatment failure.

The Internet enables this site to provide its service of information and support right across the entire globe 24 hours a day. The site provides a one-to-one mentoring service where cured individuals give ongoing support by email to those who may not be able to talk about their disease and treatment to others because of the stigma involved.

- online learning
- computer mediated learning
- computer conferencing
- virtual learning
- online learning communities
- blended learning
- learning objects
- distributed learning
- web-based learning.

All of these terms, along with the term e-learning itself, refer to the use of computer and Internet-based technologies to deliver a broad range of learning opportunities that are designed to enhance your knowledge, skills and performance. These learning opportunities are **networked**. This means that they are available via a computer connection (usually the Internet) accessible to more than one person at the same time. They, therefore, allow storage, retrieval and sharing of information and learning material – giving students and their tutors access to learning materials and communication within the learning community 24 hours a day from any Internet-connected computer on the globe. Learning opportunities are delivered to the learner via a computer that uses standard Internet technology and it focuses on the broadest views of learning that go beyond traditional approaches (Rosenberg 2001). It is about much more than the delivery of learning materials, but about a new approach to the facilitation of learning (see Box 1.2).

Box 1.2

E-learning scenarios
Here are two scenarios that highlight the differences between traditional approaches to learning and e-learning.

Traditional learning delivery
Helen is a qualified health/social care professional who works with children in a small town. She has been qualified for some years and is thinking of seeking promotion. She decides to enrol on a course to update her knowledge and skills in the area of practice in which she works. She enrols on a course at her local university – it is broadly relevant to the work that she does and she feels confident that it should help her to move forward in her practice. The course takes two years and will mean that she needs to attend lectures and seminars at the university for one day a week during semester time. She has access to experienced and knowledgeable teaching staff, the library where she can borrow books and a variety of other resources that are available both on the campus and through the university website. This means that Helen needs to be released from her workplace on a regular day each week and travel 25 miles from her home to the university.

E-learning delivery
Joanne is also a qualified health/social care practitioner who works with children in a different small town. Joanne is also thinking about extending her knowledge and skills, but she wants to make certain that she undertakes a programme that is entirely relevant to her practice with children with life-threatening conditions. Her local university provides courses that are broadly relevant, but she feels that she would benefit from a more specialist course. Following a search on the Internet she discovers that a university 150 miles away provides a course that is exactly what she is looking for. Fortunately, the course is delivered online via e-learning, so in spite of her concerns that she has not learnt in this way before, she decides to enrol. Joanne is provided with a tutor to guide her through the e-learning processes. She can contact the tutor by telephone, email or a variety of other online methods. With her fellow students, she uses a 'virtual learning environment', which she accesses via an Internet connection at home and in her workplace. The virtual learning environment provides her not only with learning materials for her reading and study, but also with communication tools so that she can discuss her thoughts, ideas and concerns with her tutor and fellow students. Because of the nature of the course, Joanne can schedule her study time to fit in with her weekly practice activity. She has found she learns best in the mornings so chooses two mornings each week in which to study online. At the beginning of the course she discovers that two of the students on the course are from another country.

E-learning has many similarities with distance learning. This is a mode of learning where the student is often some distance away, even in a different country, from the institution that provides the learning programme. The student is usually sent printed learning materials through the post and has access to a tutor via telephone and **email**. Many distance learning courses also arrange **face-to-face** tutorials and study workshops at intervals throughout the programme. E-learning is different from distance learning in the way that it uses online communication tools to maintain contact and socialization between students, their tutors and their fellow students. While distance learning does have some of the same flexibility as e-learning, it does not have the advantage of the communication options offered by online working.

Why e-learning?

There are certain features of health and social care education and practice that have led to increasing interest in e-learning as a method of delivery for education and staff development.

First, health and social care organizations employ large numbers of people with varied backgrounds and roles. For example, did you know that in the United Kingdom, the National Health Service (NHS) employs more people than any other organization in the country? This means that, in order to keep its staff well educated and well informed, the organizations involved have to be well organized and effective in the delivery of education and staff development. Economies of scale and organization are a very important consideration.

Next, the nature of health and social care practice is led by patients and clients. These are people in need of effective assessment, support and intervention in a variety of health and social care settings. Health and social care take place in a constantly changing environment where new knowledge and ideas are impacting on practice, education and management on a daily basis. The need, therefore, for the staff that work in these organizations to be well educated, up to date and highly skilled is paramount. Health and social care professionals need to communicate with each other, not just locally but globally, in order to ensure that innovative ideas, new trends and effective practice are shared amongst the practice community. The logistics of keeping large numbers of professionals with common goals in touch with each other are considered one of the major challenges of health and social care practice today and this can have a great impact on the experience of the patient or client.

As online courses and materials become increasingly available, interactive and innovative health and social care workers will be able to work through problem-solving simulations of practice situations so that they are able to see the consequences of their actions, choices and the decisions they make. This enables practitioners to learn about situations and actions in a safe environment by learning from their mistakes (Dawes and Handscomb 2002). An example of this in health care is in emergency trauma care where an activity called moulage is used to simulate and role play emergency situations and learners can make decisions about management options while receiving feedback. An example of such an activity can be found at http://www.trauma. org/resus/moulage/moulage.html (see Figure 1.1). Another perceived benefit for the empowerment of patients and clients is the potential for technology and Internet-based materials and communications to enable patients and clients to access information, enabling them to self-manage short- and long-term conditions. Such technology also allows the development of online communities of support for both patients and carers (NHS National Workforce Group 2005). An example of this is online support groups for sufferers of depression at http://www.dbsalliance.org/Info/supportgroups.html.

Much health and social care practice takes place across a 24-hour period. Many practitioners who work in these settings work at different hours of the day and night. In addition, patient and client demand means that it is not always possible for practitioners to leave the workplace on a specified day at a specified time. Indeed, most of the world now lives in what we call a 24-hour culture where we are able to access services and entertainment 24 hours a day.

Whether we like it or not, health and social care provision is, to a large degree, governed by costs and this is unlikely to change as the twenty-first

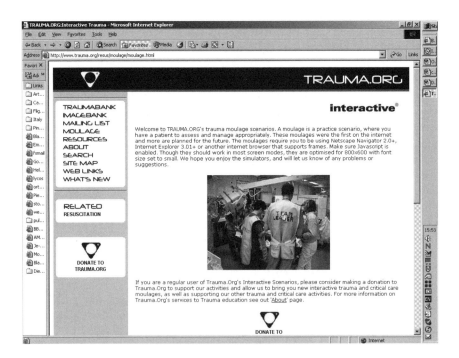

Figure 1.1 Front page of the moulage pages from www.trauma.org

century unfolds. Health and social care are very expensive 'businesses' to run, no matter where in the world they are. The need for staff education and professional development to be cost-effective is extremely important and providers are constantly looking for ways to keep the relevant budget in check.

It is with these issues in mind that both health and social care bodies have begun to consider the use of e-learning for the delivery of education for their practitioners. Here are some examples of statements from both health and social care government documents:

> within a societal context where e-government and e-society are major planks of government policy that include reference to wired up communities, wired up services and e-learning. The incorporation of e-learning is now an expected part of the student learning experience. The evidence base for e-learning shows it can be used to enhance the student programme experience and has both strengths and limitations. E-learning and communication and information technologies offer a wide range of opportunities to support development of effective, efficient and flexible open, distance and on demand learning; access to knowledge and evidence based legislation and guidance.
>
> (Rafferty and Waldman 2003)

> Developing e-learning awareness and capability covering the use of new (electronic) technologies will be essential to support open and on-line learning processes. The Internet and email are a daily part of everyday life for millions of people and businesses and knowledge management technology is rapidly being adopted by many organizations. The national vision for learning for the NHS is to enable staff to access learning opportunities at times and places that best fit in with their lifestyle. This means 24-hour access to knowledge and learning resources, 365 days per year from places that are most convenient for individuals and groups, with the technical support and structure to ensure this happens.
>
> (Department of Health (DoH) 2001)

There are many reasons why health and social care staff would wish to engage in e-learning (see Activity 1.1). The main benefits are likely to be linked to flexibility of study in time and place.

Lifelong learning

Lifelong learning is central to the government's policies for education (DfES 2006) and it is also instrumental in education strategies for health and social care (DoH 2001). The principles of lifelong learning acknowledge that, in a rapidly changing world in which knowledge is constantly moving, initial qualification and registration are not sufficient to maintain the currency of the knowledge of health and social care practitioners. Skills and knowledge,

Activity 1.1

Your reasons

We have outlined above some of the reasons why e-learning is of benefit to health and social care organizations. More important, however, are your reasons for deciding to investigate the possibilities of e-learning. Think about the reasons why you have picked up this book and try to identify five of them below:

1 _____
   _____

2 _____
   _____

3 _____
   _____

4 _____
   _____

5 _____
   _____

therefore, need to be continually refreshed and updated according to the needs and demands of the role a health or social care practitioner undertakes (Haigh 2004). The need to be constantly engaging in education, therefore, is a central tenet of the need for flexible modes of learning that can fit in with the working day and the practitioner's lifestyle. In addition health (Glenn and Cox 2006: 9) and social care staff require demonstrated competence in using common software packages such as **word processing**, email, **spreadsheets** and **databases** as well as being able to access literature and use patient and client computerized information systems (see Activity 1.2).

It could also be argued that there are more personal reasons for health and social care practitioners to engage in lifelong learning. The main reason many professionals engage in learning activity is to provide them with added interest and motivation in their work and to give them the opportunity to learn with others with similar interests. Professionals who are constantly updating their knowledge often perceive that they have enhanced job satisfaction because their view of their work is constantly changing and they are improving their effectiveness. The rewards for this often come from feedback from clients, patients and carers and from the personal satisfaction of knowing that a good job was done that made a difference to someone's life – after all, this is often the reason why individuals have chosen health or social care careers. In addition to this, it is said that managers often perceive practitioners who

Activity 1.2

Your lifelong learning

Think about yourself as a newly qualified practitioner or new student:

- What did you not know about your practice then that you know now?
- What new and enhanced skills have you since gained?
- What other skills are required for you to practise effectively now?
- What skills and knowledge might help to further your career?
- What plans do you have for your future career that will involve demonstrating a commitment to a deeper level of learning about some aspects of your practice?

engage in lifelong learning as more proactive and motivated, and this is likely to lead to job enhancement and promotion.

Communities of practice

In an increasingly **globalized** professional community and knowledge arena (Holt et al. 2000) many believe that e-learning is a way to bring many learners together into **communities of practice**. An online community of practice is a group of professional practitioners, often from the same or related professional background, who come together to share ideas and experiences, to learn and to tackle professional and work-based problems and issues (Lewis and Allan 2005: 6). Online communities of practice allow individuals who are geographically disparate to come together online rather than face-to-face – thus making the process much more flexible. Mutual engagement in activities related to a common interest allows members of a community to work together towards a common goal. Students can engage in interprofessionally based discussion that are promoted by an initial trigger and relate to elements of their academic work (Moule 2006: 43) These issues will be explored in more detail in Chapter 8.

E-learning communities

E-learning can be delivered and supported entirely using electronic media, but it can be mixed with face-to-face and other more traditional components such as lectures or seminars. This is known as **blended learning**. An example might be a course where some of the learning is sought through classroom-based formats such as lecturers or face-to-face tutorials and other aspects are delivered online or in electronic format. In some instances such as the learning of clinical skills, learning just has to take place face-to-face, of course.

It is important to remember that e-learning is much more than just **logging on** and reading something or working through an online or **CD-Rom multimedia** package. It's a whole new interactive process that may involve working with reading and other learning materials but is really based on online discussion with fellow students and tutors: 'Tell me, and I will forget. Show me and I may remember. Involve me, and I will understand' (Confucius 450 BCE).

Many educators would argue that traditional education settings such as lecture theatres and classrooms are not always the best environments in which to facilitate learning. That approach assumes that students' brains are empty vessels waiting to be filled up with knowledge directly from the mouth of the teacher or lecturer (Forman et al. 2002). There is an argument that says that the best kind of learning is that in which the student has taken an active part and that best suits their style of learning. This is the basis on which distance and open learning have been developed in the past. E-learning is really a modern extension of such approaches.

For learners like you, e-learning provides many potential benefits. Some of these are:

- flexibility in time and space – limited only by access to the Internet
- a fun, different way to learn
- the ability to study at home without having to travel to a classroom
- the opportunity to work with other students and tutors online who are too far away to meet face to face
- a student-centred approach to learning that allows the student to learn at their own pace at a time that best suits their lives
- learning that builds on the student's prior learning.

This is all very much in keeping with the current drive for lifelong learning – which encourages everyone to be active in seeking learning to support his or her professional and personal lives.

However, there are a few things we need to consider that might be the pitfalls of e-learning:

- There is a danger that, because of the flexibility of e-learning, insufficient time is laid aside for studies. Your manager or workplace supervisor might believe, for example, that because you can study at any time of the day or night they might not need to provide you with official study leave. This is very far from the case. Equally, your own view of the time you expect to devote to your studies is very important.
- Not everyone has access to the technology required. Not everyone has an Internet connection at home and those who do may not have a **broadband** Internet connection that provides the most efficient access to the Internet. Equally, although health and social care organizations are working

towards a good level of Internet access in the workplace, cost constraints and the nature of the workplace means that it will still be some time before this becomes a reality.

- Many potential e-learning students do not consider themselves to have the technical skills required to access learning. Computer skills vary considerably between individuals and many professionals feel uncomfortable about using computers and the Internet. Even though only basic computer skills are required for e-learning – the need to access the Internet can still be a source of fear and anxiety for many students and potential students.

- Not being aware of the time and effort involved in an e-learning course is a major issue for students setting out as e-learners for the first time. We have found that students are quite shocked by the amount of effort they must put in. E-learning is a very rewarding form of learning that means the student takes responsibility for what they are learning while receiving the right amount of support from their tutors. It also means that it is impossible for you to leave all your active learning activity until the end of the course, programme or module as in other approaches to learning. There are specific tasks and activities to undertake that are designed to space your learning out and keep it on track. This is thought to help most people to learn more effectively. It means that it's very difficult to sit back for the first half of the module and do very little and then 'cram' in all your learning at the end. Assessments and assignments for e-learning students are often designed so that you have to demonstrate you have worked all the way through the module. You will find that you have to start reading and writing from week one. If you need to be organized, this might be an advantage for you.

Widening participation

Many educational institutions expect or hope that online learning will make learning available to users who would otherwise be unable to participate away from the traditional pool of possible students. This includes an international market as well as more local ones. Not only does this enable students from different cultural backgrounds to work together in online learning communities, but also it removes some of the difficulties of attending a face-to-face session. Disabled students, including those with a learning disability, can be enabled to learn through the use of learning technology. Online messages appear as an individual's thoughts and are less likely to be about their age, gender, appearance or disability. Online working, for example, can open doors for those with restricted mobility (Salmon 2003: 115) or, for example, with sight or hearing impairments. If you have any kind of disability, it is worth talking to your chosen education institution, which will most likely have a tutor who specializes in this area. It is helpful to find out what facilities are on offer for you as a student to support you in this new learning environment.

Conclusion

E-learning is a relatively new and exciting way of learning for health and social care practitioners. E-learning has a number of benefits to health and social care practice, but these can be reaped only if the right mechanisms and facilities are in place for students including a place and the time to learn. It provides students with a stimulating approach to learning that is more self-led than other students.

References

ComScore (2006) http://www.comscore.com/press/release.asp?press=849 (accessed 24 August 2006).

Dawes, D. and Handscomb, A. (2002) A pilot study to assess the case for e-learning in the NHS. *NT Research* 7 (6): 428–443.

Department for Education and Skills (2005) *Harnessing Technology: Transforming Learning and Children's Services*. London: DfES. Available at http://www.dfes.gov.uk/publications/e-strategy (accessed 24 August 2006).

Department for Education and Skills (2006) Available at www.lifelonglearning.co.uk (accessed 24 August 2006).

Department of Health (2001) *Working Together – Learning Together: A Framework for Lifelong Learning in the NHS*. London: Department of Health. Available at: http://www.dh.gov.uk/PublicationsAndStatistics/Publications/PublicationsPolicyAndGuidance/PublicationsPolicyAndGuidanceArticle/fs/en?CONTENT_ID=4009558&chk=tCWmaW (accessed 24 August 2006).

Forman, D., Nyatanga, L. and Rich, T. (2002) E-learning and educational diversity. *Nurse Education Today* 22 (1): 76–82.

Glenn, S. and Cox, H. (2006) E-learning in nursing: the context. In: Glenn, S. and Moule, P. (eds) *E-learning in Nursing*. Chapter 1. Basingstoke: Palgrave.

Haigh, J. (2004) Information technology in health professional education: why IT matters. *Nurse Education Today* 24 (7): 547–552.

Holt, J., Barrett, C., Clarke, D. and Monks, R. (2000) The globalization of nursing knowledge. *Nurse Education Today* 20 (6): 426–431.

Lewis, D. and Allan B. (2005) *Virtual Learning Communities: A Guide for Practitioners*. Maidenhead: The Society for Research into Higher Education and Open University Press.

Moule, P. (2006) E-communities. In: Glenn, S. and Moule, P. (eds) *E-learning in Nursing*. Chapter 3. Basingstoke: Palgrave.

NHS National Workforce Group (2005) *Supporting Best Practice in E-learning across the NHS*. Available at: http://www.informatics.nhs.uk/download/2094/national_strategy.pdf (accessed 24 August 2006).

Rafferty, J. and Waldman, J. (2003) *Building Capacity to Support the Social Work Degree: A Scoping Study for the Department of Health Elearning Steering Group*. London: Department of Health. Available at http://www.practicelearning.org.uk/downloads/5.pdf (accessed 24 August 2006).

Rosenberg, M.J. (2001) *E-learning – Strategies for Delivering Knowledge in the Digital Age*. New York: McGraw-Hill.

Salmon, G. (2003) *E-moderating: The Key to Online Learning and Teaching*. London: Routledge Falmer.

Recommended further reading

Clark, A. (2004) *E-learning Skills*. Basingstoke: Palgrave.

Chellen, S.S. (2003) *The Essential Guide to the Internet for Health Professionals*. London: Routledge.

Lewis, D. and Allan, B. (2005) *Virtual Learning Communities: A Guide for Practitioners*. Maidenhead: The Society for Research into Higher Education and Open University Press.

2 Skills for successful online learning

Introduction

The aim of this chapter is to help you to focus on your own learning processes and styles and existing learning skills and to help you to adapt them for e-learning. The chapter will include an opportunity for you to think about your own readiness to learn as an online learner both in terms of your practical ability and readiness and in relation to your motivation. Practical advice will be given on how to improve such readiness and how you might develop additional skills should this be required. Some of this will involve the development of your technical skills. The important thing to recognize is that many of the skills you already have as a learner will be of great use to you and the need for technical skills is relatively small.

Being an e-learner involves self-directedness in ways that do not always apply to other learning methods. Many health and social care students study part time and need to balance busy lives as practitioners with their studies as well as home life. It is essential that time management is considered a major issue in successful learning.

The role of reflection and supervision and how these can be transferred to the online environment will be illuminated. We will also include a brief discussion of the practical application of **constructivism** to online learning from a student support perspective. You will also be offered advice on how to develop your computer and technical skills. Skills in the application of theory to practice alongside evidence-based practice will be discussed. Finally, this chapter includes some advice on how to seek support for learning difficulties, such as dyslexia.

Being an e-learner – computer access and skills

In order to be a successful online learner it is essential that you have access to an Internet-connected computer. It is essential that this access is uninterrupted and available at times that you need to access it. It must also be at a location that is conducive to studying. It's no use trying to study on a home computer that is in a part of the house that is open to constant interruption by other members of the household (including the dog or cat!) or in a busy **Internet café**. Nor is it helpful to use a computer in the workplace that is being used for other purposes at the same time and is located in an area in which there is a lot of noisy and distracting activity. You need to think very carefully about whether you have adequate *local* computer access. It may be necessary for you to investigate using a computer at your local library, for example, if you are unable to access a computer of your own or, at the very least, one to which you have uninterrupted access at the right time. It is worth checking with your education institution whether they have any reciprocal arrangements with institutions nearer you for you to use their computer systems or suites. If you don't currently own a computer, now is probably a good time to think about buying your first one. Most universities and colleges now have excellent access to computers for their students – often placed in a variety of areas across a campus or within a building. Even though the whole purpose of e-learning is to be able to work remotely, this may be the only option for you. If you are studying with such an organization, these computers are free to use for all students and will be the most economical way of accessing a computer if you don't have one at home. To take advantage of this you need to find out, very early on, before your course starts exactly where these computers are located and the opening hours, as well as how the log-in systems work. All universities and colleges will have **user names** and **passwords** that protect their systems from use by those who don't have a right to use them. Clearly, it is essential that you have access on day one of your course, so you will need to make sure that you have registered and been given your access codes and passwords. Delays in this are likely to make you struggle at the beginning of the course just when you need to be getting used to it.

In addition to the computer itself, you also need a reliable Internet connection, preferably high-speed broadband. This is important because you are likely to need to **download** materials such as large documents and **digital** video from the Internet and you need the facilities to do this quickly. There are two ways of connecting to the Internet. The first uses a normal telephone line to dial a number for the Internet provider. This is known as **dial-up** access. This is now considered a rather slow and inefficient way to access the Internet. Broadband access, on the other hand, uses a different kind of channel (although it often uses a telephone line initially) that accesses and downloads information much more quickly.

You will also need some basic technical skills. All of the computer skills required of an e-learner are those expected of the average person in the workplace nowadays. A computer-literate workforce that is able to seek information and communicate using the Internet is seen by many as essential to the optimum development of health (Haigh 2004) and social care. The ability to undertake basic tasks is necessary for engagement in everyday life. It is no longer possible for the student or employee to ignore the need to develop basic computer skills.

Box 2.1 is a checklist of the most essential computer access and skills needed for the e-learner.

If you do have these skills – you already have some of the tools you need to be a successful e-learner! If you have some of them, the checklist should help you to work out which ones you need to work on. If you don't have any, you may need to attend a basic computer skills course or a study skills course prior to commencing an e-learning course. Many local colleges now provide computer skills courses right from the basic to more advanced. It is worth considering attending a course that provides the **European Computer Driving Licence (ECDL)** (or similar) course that will give you all the basic skills you need to use a computer and its **software package** as well as an internationally recognized qualification. No prior knowledge of IT or computer skills are needed for the beginners' courses. You can get more information on this from, among others, your local further education provider or library, or from www.ecdl.co.uk. You should also look out for study skills courses provided by your local education providers specifically for health and social care students. These are more likely to fit your needs in terms of helping you to learn how to access relevant good quality information in your subject area. Your university or college may also provide free basic computer courses and it is a good idea to see if you can access these before your **online** course begins. See also Box 2.2.

In addition to these more self-directed approaches, your e-learning tutor should be able to help. Tutors are well aware that students need support in

---

Box 2.1

A checklist of computer essentials for e-learners

- Having a personal email account either at home or at work or both.
- Having uninterrupted access to an Internet-connected computer.
- Being able to send and receive emails with **attachments**.
- Being able to use a word processing package such as Microsoft Word to produce simple text documents.
- Being able to search for, access and navigate around **websites** on relevant subject areas, and to critically appraise the material offered – this is often known as **surfing** the web.
- Being able to use **electronic databases** to search for learning materials (such as journal articles) in subject areas specific to the student's area of study.
- Being able to manage files on the computer and save and back-up your work and other information.
- Having the facility to print documents as needed (see p. 29).

Box 2.2

BBC 'My Web My Way'

In addition to the suggestions in this chapter, help can be found at a variety of places on the Internet itself. One example is the 'My Web My Way' service from the BBC at: http://www.bbc.co.uk/accessibility (accessed 24 August 2006).

This site provides help in making the Web easier to use. It explains the many ways you can change your browser, computer, keyboard and mouse settings to make the Web more accessible for you according to your needs. It is fairly simple to use, so we recommend that you pay it a visit.

using online systems, especially in the early weeks of a course. Your tutor will help you to get started if you need it. The most important thing is to be honest with your tutor about what previous experience you have of working online and with computers, and to let them know immediately if you are having problems. Some students feel embarrassed about the gaps in their computer skills and tutors are very aware that this is likely to be the case. Many students are anxious about the technological aspects of being an e-learner, but they usually pick it up very quickly once they get started. You will find out more about the support you can expect from the e-tutor in Chapter 4.

Your learning style

Adult learners vary in the way that they prefer to learn. They will often have developed their own approach to learning over the years since childhood. You will have developed your own approaches during your life. Many of us have our own preferred approach to learning, for example:

- Some prefer to learn alone while others prefer to learn in groups.
- Many people prefer to learn from doing rather than watching or listening.
- People approach the process of reading and note taking in many different ways.

Rarely do we actually think about the way in which we learn. Before you embark on an e-learning course, it is a good idea to assess your learning styles and to think about your attitudes to learning and the approaches you take. Think about some of the questions in Activity 2.1.

Thinking about some of the issues raised in Activity 2.1 will help you to identify some of the processes that you use for learning (see Activity 2.2).

Activity 2.1

Your learning style

Think about the following questions:

1 Do you prefer to listen to a lecture rather than read material in a book or journal in order to learn?
2 Do you like to have things explained to you, beginning with simple explanations and moving on to the more complex approach?
3 Do you prefer visual information or aural information?
4 When you were a classroom student, did you tend to participate freely in discussions or did you tend to listen more to what others have to say?
5 Do you make notes from lectures and your reading, and review them later?
6 Do you find that the pace of classroom sessions or lectures is often either too slow or too fast for you?

Activity 2.2

Learning styles

Undertake an Internet search (for example, try using Google at www.google.co.uk) using the search terms 'learning styles' and 'e-learning'. (If you need help with conducting an Internet search there is more help in this chapter and in Chapter 5.) Explore a few of the websites that the search tool offers you. You will probably find some that offer you the opportunity to complete an online learning style questionnaire and get feedback on your learning style for free.

Write down some of the things you find that illuminate your own learning style/s:

You will find that most 'study skills' books will offer you some advice about how to think about and adapt your learning style. There are also a number of study skills websites that will also help you with this, for example: www.how-to-study.com.

Because students have so many different learning styles, not all fit every learning situation. What is important is that you recognize where your learning style fits e-learning and where it doesn't, so that you can identify strategies for dealing with this. Box 2.3 has an example.

Motivation

In Chapter 1 we looked briefly at your reasons for wanting to be an e-learner. Motivation is a central skill in successful learning generally, but it is even more central in all forms of self-directed learning such as e-learning. When you undertake an online course, your motivation is not driven by attending regular lectures and physically being with your tutor and other students. You are generally more free to organize your learning according to your own needs

---

Box 2.3

Josie's learning style

Josie is an experienced social care professional who decided she wanted to do an advanced course in her area of specialist expertise. The course she most wanted to do was at a university some miles away, but it was offered as an online option, so she felt that this may still meet her needs. She wasn't sure how she would get along with online learning as she had never done it before, so she decided to undertake a short e-learning module at her local university to give her an idea of how it might work for her.

One of the first things she did on the course was to look at her personal learning style in more detail. She discovered that she was definitely someone who liked to work with others. She also discovered that she liked to be able to see those she was working with face to face. Because of this she, initially, found the online nature of the module quite difficult. She never got to meet her tutor or her fellow students face to face and she was quite uncomfortable with this at the beginning. Gradually, though, she 'got to know' her tutor and the other students as the online discussions developed and she started to build up a picture of the people she was working with. This really helped and she found that she took to this way of communicating and learning by the end of the module. She had a lot of really good support from the tutor, who seemed to recognize that she and the other students might find this difficult. She decided to apply for the other course. She felt that her learning style didn't suit online working perfectly, but that she was prepared to make some adjustments in order to make it work for her.

and desires. The motivation to learn in e-learning is largely intrinsic and comes from within the learner rather than extrinsic motivation in which the student is driven by external sources. This can be quite disorientating for those who are used to external drivers. It is essential that you consider not only what motivates you to learn, but also how you will bridge any gaps in that motivation. The online 'classroom' is very different from the traditional classroom approach and will present you with a variety of obstacles, dilemmas and opportunities that you will need to overcome and make the best of. The student needs strong motivation and encouragement to put in the necessary time and effort to learn successfully (Salmon 2003). Unless you are committed to learning in the first place you are unlikely to be able to sustain this motivation (see Activity 2.3).

Activity 2.3

Adjustments

Think about what 'adjustments' (things in your life you might need to change or give up for a while to make room for your studies) you might need to make in your life in order to fit e-learning into your schedule. Write five of them down below.

Score them from zero to five in terms of how important they are to you (zero is no importance and five is the highest level of importance possible) and score them again in terms of how much you are willing to make sacrifices in order to give you time to learn (zero is no willingness to sacrifice and five is total willingness). Be honest and positive in your approach.

Think about how your willingness to sacrifice (or not) some of the things in your life might affect your progress as an e-learner.

Adjustments	Importance (0–5)	Willingness to sacrifice (0–5)
1		
2		
3		
4		
5		

Time management

In our experience, students are often quite surprised by the amount of time they have to devote to their studies as an e-learner. Some students even become a little 'addicted' to logging-on and finding out what has been happening in the **discussion boards** and **chat rooms**. Because of the flexibility of this mode of learning, students often mistakenly feel that it is likely to be less time consuming. This is not the case. E-learners are committed to a way of learning that includes regular involvement in an online community and this takes considerable effort and time. Your e-learning tutor should be able to give you an idea of how much time, on average, is needed each week in order to learn successfully, but this will be only a rough figure and you may find you need to commit more or less time, depending on how you learn.

It is important to remember that this is a very different way of learning and it will take some time and effort to get used to it, so you may find it more time consuming in the beginning.

There are two aspects to the time involved in learning online:

- The time needed to log on and participate in any online discussions and chats that might be happening as well as to pick up instructions from your tutors about the learning activities you need to undertake.
- The time needed to undertake the learning activities that will enable you to participate in online discussions effectively. This might be an activity that involves searching for information, or reading a specific paper or a thinking task. These are sometimes known as **e-tivities** (Salmon 2002).

For example, you might need to log on at the beginning of the week to find out about a new activity and then come back later in the week to discuss your learning with the other students. Organizing time to undertake both of these sets of activities is really important. It is a good idea to set aside time every two days or so to enable you to keep your learning fresh in your mind and participate actively in online activities and discussions. Set aside time as if you were actually attending a class. It is all too easy to think 'Oh, I'm an e-learner, e-learning is flexible, I can do it any time, I'll just fit it in between all the other things I have to do in my life.' This is a recipe for failure. You need to set regular time aside and get into the habit of sticking to it. It is also a good idea to spread what time you have available over the week, but not in such short stretches that you can't get into what you need to do – three periods of 1.5 hours often works well for many. If you are a full-time student or undertaking a more intensive course of study, you need to think realistically about exactly how much time your course will need (see Activity 2.4).

Being organized is central to good study practice. It is particularly important in e-learning as there will be lots of information stored in lots of different places both electronically and on paper that you will need to refer to. It is often the case that these pieces of information will be needed to

Activity 2.4

Time to study

Write down the days of the week and times you are most likely to be able to set time aside for learning.

Add up the numbers of hours per week this would involve

Do you think this will be enough for you to learn what you need? Is it realistic?

Put these slots into your diary or onto your calendar and then stick to them. If you don't normally keep a diary, now is the time to consider getting one.

construct the assessment for your course and that you will want to refer back to them later.

One good idea is to keep a **learning journal**. You can use this for two purposes:

- to enable you to write down your thoughts and reflections on your learning experience
- to make notes about the things you want to remember for future reference.

Data storage

Importantly, you need to think about storage of **data** (pieces of information you may need to refer back to at a later date). These need to be placed somewhere you can find them easily and where they won't get lost.

The first step is to make sure that you have all electronic files in a safe and accessible place. These files will include reading materials and any work that you have done. There are a number of places you can store these:

- On your computer **hard drive** – this is a large electronic data storage compartment in your computer – it's often also known as the 'C: Drive'. It will allow you to store and retrieve a large number of files. You must store the files in folders and sub-folders, a bit like in a filing cabinet to enable you to find them easily.
- On **disks**. These are portable forms of data storage. There are a number of different types of these. You can save files to a **floppy disk** – which are the smallest kind of data storage that tend to operate from the 'A: Drive' in your computer. The alternatives are **compact discs** (CDs) that look like music CDs and have a much larger capacity. CDs quite often need a

special software package to allow you to save (or burn) data onto them and some are non-rewritable in that once data is stored on them it can't be wiped and replaced. Floppy disks and CDs are quite cheap to buy these days.

- One popular way of storing data these days is on a **USB flash drive** or 'memory stick'. These are small, portable devices that are often smaller than a marker-pen. These connect directly into a port on your computer known as a USB port. The advantages of these are that they carry large amounts of data on a very small and light piece of equipment that can be carried in your pocket. These are more expensive, but are getting cheaper and are very convenient.
- Some colleges and universities will also offer you the opportunity to save your files to a large 'hard drive' in the university itself. The advantage of this is that your files are accessible from any networked computer in the university and the files are usually backed up at least once a day so that if anything goes wrong the files can be retrieved from the back-up.

This brings us on to a very important point about backing up files. Computer disks, whatever the kind, can go wrong and data can be lost. For this reason it is vital that you make AT LEAST ONE copy of your files, certainly those which are important to you, so that if your work is lost or **corrupted**, you can retrieve it from another source. This is probably one of the most important tips in this book! It is now no longer acceptable to tell your tutor your work is late because your computer broke down (or **crashed**) and you have lost all your work.

Another word of caution revolves around the files that you create and/or share with other students in the **virtual learning environment** (VLE) in which you work. It is important that these systems are designed for data *sharing* and not data *storage*. To this end, if you are sharing files with other students in a section of the VLE, do not assume that they will always be there and make sure that you keep a copy of the file on your own computer or on a portable disc.

An important aspect of studying is referencing your written work with your reading. Advice about this can be found on the Internet, in your university and college handbooks and guidance and in study skills books. Keeping track of these references when you are producing large pieces of work such as assignments and theses can be quite difficult. Some students like to use databases and other specially designed software that enables them to keep track of their reading and references. These are known as 'personal bibliographic management tools' and they help the individual student or researcher to record, organize and use citations of references to sources of information – predominantly articles and books – used in the course of their work. Some examples of these tools are EndNote (www.endnote.com), ProCite (www.procite.com) and Reference Manager (www.refman.com).

Printing

During your online course of study you will access and collect a wide variety of digital written material. There is a danger that you will print out everything for later referral. This can be an expensive strategy. If you print out everything you think appears useful at first sight, it is almost guaranteed that you will go back to read only about 10 per cent of it. Most people prefer to read from the printed word, but taking a print-and-read-later approach means that you will use large amounts of printer ink and paper, which is unnecessary and can prove expensive. Our advice is to save everything you think you want to come back to into files and folders that you will be able to find again later. This way you can go back and review the material when you need it again and be certain that you print out only that which you are certain you will need to use for your studies.

Downloading

One of the ways in which you will access learning material is by downloading it (accessing material from the Internet and saving it as a file on your own computer) from **websites** and **VLEs**. The kind of material you need to download will vary from video and audio material that you can watch and listen to online, to files that contain reading material such as journal articles and materials produced by your tutors. Many of these files will be available in what is known as **Portable Document Format file (PDF file)**. These files are created using software that packages the file in a way that is easy to load onto Internet pages, but can only be read, and not altered, by the person who has downloaded it. In order to download and read these files you will need specific software – most computers come ready loaded with this software, but you may need to access the software from the Internet and save it to your computer, especially if the software is out of date.

The most common software for creating PDF files converts the files into formats readable using Adobe Acrobat Reader. This is free software that can be downloaded for no charge at http://www.adobe.com/products/acrobat/readstep2.html. You just need to click on the download button and follow the online instructions.

Some files will also be available to you in what is known as **HTML** format. HTML is a term for the language that your computer uses to make material readable from and on the Internet. Files available in HTML do not need any specific software other than a **web browser** to open them and they take up less memory because they are in a simpler format.

In addition, your tutors may have created files for you to view in presentation creation software known as Microsoft **PowerPoint**®. Many students' computers do not come loaded with this software, so it may be difficult for you to download the files. Microsoft offers a free 'PowerPoint Reader' that can also be downloaded from http://www.microsoft.com/downloads.

Email

Email is an increasing feature of everyday life both at work and at home. Email is mail that is composed and transmitted on a computer system or network almost instantly. It has revolutionized the way in which people communicate with each other and stay in touch across the globe because it is a fast, cheap and effective way of communicating between individuals who may be great distances apart. It takes no longer to send an email from London, England to Sydney, Australia than it does to someone in the next room.

Everyone who uses email has a unique address. An email address is made up of several parts. The first part of the address, the username, identifies a unique user on a computer server. The @ symbol separates the username from the host name. The host name uniquely identifies the server computer and is the last part of the Internet email address. The three-letter suffix in the host name identifies the kind of organization operating the server. The most common suffixes are: .com (commercial), .edu (educational), .gov (government), .mil (military), .net (networking) and .org (non-commercial), but new ones are becoming increasingly available. Final two-letter suffixes generally identify a geographical area: .uk (United Kingdom), .de (Germany), .ca (Canada), etc. As an example, our email addresses use our names and indicate that the host address is from a university in the United Kingdom:

J.Santy@hull.ac.uk
M.E.Smith@hull.ac.uk

Email is used in commercial organizations for communications internally and externally. It is used in health and social care organizations to allow staff to communicate with one another and to disseminate information to large numbers of individuals at once. It can also be used to add attachments to messages. This is where documents and photographs (which the recipient can then download onto their own computer) can be sent along with a message. This is particularly useful when more than one individual needs to work on those files from a distance. Email is, therefore, an extremely useful communication tool to enable you to contact your tutor and fellow students on e-learning courses.

One of the biggest problems with email is what is known as **spam** or **junk mail**. This is the unsolicited, unwanted, irrelevant or inappropriate sending of emails in mass quantities, commonly as an advertising ploy. This is a nuisance and often uses up lots of computer memory. Many organizations are working on systems to reduce spam. The other problem is the large volumes of emails generated in some organizations, causing email **inboxes** to become clogged up. This can be a major issue in health and social care organizations.

There are, however, many advantages to using email:

- Emails are usually delivered almost instantly, within moments of sending, no matter where in the world they are sent. This makes for spontaneous communication.

- Emailing as a form of communication is very cheap once you have an Internet connection. Many Internet and other providers now supply email systems at no cost to non-commercial individuals and organizations.
- You can usually access your email messages from any Internet-connected computer on the globe, meaning that you can stay in touch wherever you can access a computer.
- Email can be paperless, so it is perceived as being environmentally friendly.
- Email is also seen to negate the need for some telephone conversations.

Email is an exceptionally useful e-learning tool. It allows individuals to send and receive personal messages containing important information. In the case of many e-learning courses, initial instructions for joining the course will be sent by email, and this will be followed by further information sent via this route. It enables large and frequent communication without the worry of distance. It is, therefore, absolutely vital that you have an active email address and you are able to access and respond to these easily.

Your email skills

In order to use email effectively you will need to be able to do the following:

- Set up and log in to an email account. Email accounts will generally be provided free for you by your place of employment or education institution and both of these will provide you with instructions on how to use the system. If you have an Internet provider at home, they will also provide you with an email account. If this is not the case, or if you want to explore your own options, there are many Internet providers who will provide you with free email and their sites contain help on how to do so. Some of the more common examples are:
- MSN Hotmail: http://join.msn.com/hotmail/
  Yahoo mail: http://mail.yahoo.com/
  Lycos mail: http://mail.lycos.com/
  Wanadoo: http://www.wanadoo.co.uk/communicate/email/
- Choose a suitable email address. Most email account providers will give you a degree of flexibility with this when you first set up your email account. However, it is important that you choose an email address that it is not too difficult to remember and that you won't be embarrassed to give to anyone!
- Access your email box remotely from both your home and work computers as well as others.
- Access your inbox, retrieve and open emails that have been sent to you.
- Open and save attachments from your emails.
- Reply to emails that have been sent to you.
- Compose and send emails to others.

- Add file attachments such as word processed documents to your emails.
- Manage your email folders.
- Save and delete emails.

Word processing and other software

The majority of universities and colleges will now not accept hand-written work for assessment. This means that you must produce all of your written work, such as essays, reports and theses, using a word processing package. Word processing is the creation, input, editing and production of words in documents and texts by means of a computer system. Many computers now come pre-loaded with word processing software. It is important, however, that you make sure that your own word processing tools are compatible with those of your tutor and of the institution in which your tutor works. E-learning students need to send work to their tutor as an email attachment and, if your word processing package is not compatible, your tutor will not be able to read your work. The most common word processing package in use, at home and at universities and colleges, is Microsoft Word®, but it is best to check with your tutor or institution which is the most appropriate for you.

Often in e-learning situations, you'll need to work on a document with other learners or need to send a document to your tutor for comments. There are ways of recording changes made to a document which are invaluable in these situations. Microsoft Word, for example, has a function in its **Tools menu** called Track Changes that highlights the changes that one writer makes to a document so that others can see what has been added or changed (Clarke 2004: 61). Finding out how to switch on this facility is essential. Microsoft Word also allows you to add comments boxes within the text, using a similar system.

Databases and data processing software, spreadsheets and presentation software are some of the many other computer packages that may be useful to your learning. Some of these packages will already be available on your home computer, but others may need to be purchased if you have a use for them. If you are currently not confident with word processing, we suggest that you focus on that. However, students with good word processing skills may want to expand these to the use of other packages. Many libraries will lend books and manuals about these programmes with a variety of approaches from absolute beginners to improvers and experts. Books, such as those supporting ECDL (European Computer Driving Licence) courses, can also be very useful.

Your developing skills

It's worth noting that the skills you need to successfully learn online are almost an integral and essential part of everyday life these days. It's often possible to find a family member or friend who can help you to get online and make things work for you. If you can get online, find a website and navigate around it, you are most of the way there already. The secret is to admit when you don't know how to do something and be active in finding someone, sometimes known as a 'buddy', to help you do what you need to do.

Reflection

Learning though reflection and using reflective journals and professional portfolios is actively encouraged in contemporary nurse education in the United Kingdom (Gulati 2006: 25). The idea of writing down, either in paper or electronic format, however, is also likely to be of value to other students of health and social care. Keeping a reflective diary of your thoughts and ideas about the e-learning process is one possible way of keeping track of your learning.

Conclusion

As your e-learning course progresses, you will find that your online skills improve and develop as you go along. Committed e-learners often become more engaged with the technology around them, both at home and in the workplace, and find that it enriches their lives. It is important, however, to remember that e-learning is meant to be fun and learning about the technology should be part of that.

References

Clarke, A. (2004) *E-learning Skills*. Basingstoke: Palgrave.

Gulati, S. (2006) Application of new technologies: nurse education. In: Glenn, S. and Moule, P. (eds) *E-learning in Nursing*. Chapter 2. Basingstoke: Palgrave.

Haigh, J. (2004) Information technology in health professional education: why IT matters. *Nurse Education Today* 24 (7): 547–552.

Salmon, G. (2002) *E-tivities: The Key to Active Online Learning*. London: Kogan Page.

Salmon, G. (2003) *E-moderating: The Key to Teaching and Learning Online*, 2nd edition. London: Routledge Falmer.

Recommended further reading

Chellen, S.S. (2003) *The Essential Guide to the Internet for Health Professionals*, student edition. London: Routledge.

Clark, D. and Buckley, P. (2005) *The Rough Guide to the Internet*. London: Rough Guides.

Clegg, B. (2006) *Studying Using the Web*. London: Routledge Falmer.

Cottrell, S. (2003) *The Study Skills Handbook*. Basingstoke: Palgrave Macmillan.

Levine, J.R., Young, M.L. and Baroudi, C. (2005) *The Internet for Dummies*, 10th edition. New York: John Wiley.

3 The role of the student in online learning

Introduction

This chapter will help you to identify your roles and responsibilities in e-learning. It will focus on lifelong learning and self-directed working. It will also consider issues such as managing your own learning, time management and maintaining motivation. The notion of seeking peer support will also be included – in particular, issues of mentorship, preceptorship and buddying will be briefly discussed as these are distinct models of student support that have been used in health and social care for many years. It will also consider existing e-learning theory that illuminates the role of the student as well as the role of the e-tutor and technical support.

One of the main theorists in e-learning is Gilly Salmon, who worked for the Open University for some years and has researched student and tutor interaction in e-learning. The Open University in the United Kingdom is seen as a world leader in open and distance education and a leader in the use of new technologies to support students in their learning. Gilly Salmon's book *E-moderating* (Salmon 2003) is now in its second edition. In this text, Salmon talks about a five-stage model (see Figure 3.1). The model suggests that online learning is a five-step process that illuminates the role of the student as well as the role of the e-tutor (Salmon calls the e-tutor the 'e-moderator' to reflect the facilitative role of the tutor). Each step is reliant on the one before it. At each step the student has specific responsibilities alongside the e-tutor and technical support. You don't really need to understand this model in detail. What you do need to understand is that you will, generally, be starting on the bottom step of the model and that each step further is dependent on the one before it, although some moving backwards will sometimes take place in some aspects of your learning. Here are some essential principles:

- Both you and your tutors take responsibility for your learning – but the emphasis is on you and how you self-direct your own learning and learn what you need to learn.
- In order for you to be able to learn, you need to be motivated and to have access to the right computer systems.

- Once you have access and are motivated to get online you need to 'socialize' in online discussion groups or forums with your fellow students and tutor. This recognizes the fact that learning is, essentially, a social activity and that it is unlikely to be successful unless ideas can be shared and discussed with your colleagues. This stage is very important, as it can be very central in your motivation and learning success.
- Once socialization has taken place then you can begin to exchange information within the social group that has formed. This will involve tasks created and facilitated by your tutor and in which you must participate as fully as possible. This means not only that you must take responsibility for your part in the task or activity that you have been asked to complete, but also that you must undertake to collaborate and share with your fellow students.
- In the fourth stage, you will begin to construct knowledge that is relevant and meaningful to you. The knowledge you construct will be based on your own needs and experiences through an active process that is self-led. The online activity that you participate in will have been designed to help you to do this. It may be that some students do not progress beyond this stage.
- In the final stage some students will be able to use the knowledge they have gained to develop new skills and ideas regarding practice.

E-learning provides many potential benefits. Some of these are:

- flexibility in time and space limited only by Internet access
- a fun, different way to learn
- a way of learning that recognizes your previous learning and encourages you to use this in the new learning situation
- the development of online relationships with fellow students and tutors
- access to a wealth of learning resources in a digital format
- the freedom to learn what you want or need to learn.

In order to reap these benefits, your part in the learning processes must be active and with a good degree of self-led activity. E-learning makes some assumptions about you! Overall these are as follows:

- You *want* to learn.
- You are *interested* in the subject at hand.
- You are *able* to study.
- You have regular/daily *access* to an Internet-connected computer.
- You are able to *navigate* the Internet.
- You can find your way around a *website*.
- You can use a *word processor* such as Microsoft Word or similar.
- You can send and receive *emails* with or without attachments.

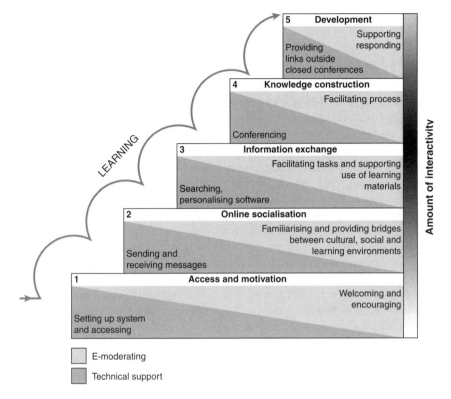

Figure 3.1 Principles of online learning: Salmon's five-stage module of teaching and learning online

Source: Salmon 2003: 29, http://www.atimod.com/e-moderating/5stage.shtml (accessed 24 August 2006)

If you are unable to say yes to each of these assumptions then you may need to do some work before you set off on your e-learning journey to make sure you are prepared. We have dealt with some of the skills you might need in more detail in Chapter 2, and it is worth reviewing any of the issues this raises for you at this stage.

Access

The ability to log on to the computer systems being used to support learning is essential. Doing this right at the beginning of the course or module is essential and, having been given instructions on how to do so, you must take full responsibility for making sure this step is made successfully. If there are problems with this access, you must also take responsibility for seeking support from the e-tutor and any technical help that is on offer. This may need to be by telephone.

Motivation and commitment

Never is motivation to learn more important than in flexible modes of learning such as e-learning, distance and open learning. E-learners and distance and open learners almost always need to work in physical isolation from their fellow students and tutors, and can not get their motivation from attending classes in a physical setting each week. Motivation must, therefore, come from within the student. E-learning is a new and exciting form of open and distance learning and, as such, interest is generated by the new and interesting ways in which e-learners communicate with each other and their tutors. However, this is related to another aspect of e-learning that makes intrinsic motivation so important. In order for e-learning to be successful, students must become part of a 'community' with their fellow students. In order to do this, e-learners must commit themselves not only to logging on to the course's website or virtual learning environment and discussion board regularly, but also to making an active contribution to that community. Much of the activity in e-learning is centred around working in online discussion forums and chat rooms with other students. If you just log on and don't contribute to the discussions, you will not find that you become part of the community. In large classrooms of students, you may be able to sit in on a discussion and just soak up what is going on – it's not so easy to do this in an online community. It's a little like moving home to a new town or village – you have to participate in the community before you can become a part of it and this needs motivation and drive to do this in the first place. If you don't make the effort you will never settle and feel at home!

Having the motivation of being 'sent' on a course is not sufficient motivation for successful learning, especially if you are to be an e-learner for the first time. In order to be committed to your e-learning course, you must find the subject matter interesting and the idea of learning about it stimulating. Your learning must be directed by your own goals. Ask yourself the following questions:

- Am I really committed to completing this course?
- What am I expecting to gain from it?
- Are those gains important to me?
- What do I expect the outcome to be?
- Am I able to set aside the time I need in order to study for this course?
- What might I need to sacrifice to be successful in achieving my goals in this course?

You may need to think carefully about these issues. Is your commitment sufficient and at the right level?

Constructivism

Constructivism is a theory of learning. You don't need to know about it in a great deal of detail, but it is worth briefly mentioning it as it explains some of the ways in which e-learning is perceived to be a good approach to learning. The theory claims that students build up their own meanings and under-standings of a topic and discover their own learning (Twomey 2004). The teacher becomes a facilitator rather than an expert and students construct their learning though putting blocks of information together in a way that is meaningful to them. This fits quite well with many approaches to online learning. Salmon (2003: 45) suggests that your construction of your own knowledge can be directly related to your interaction online with other students and this is the reason that online interaction and socialization is so important.

Socialization

Salmon (2003: 33) argues that many of the benefits of online work flow from working in an online community of people who are working together at common tasks. She says that there are two motives for people to work together – self-interest and common interest. Working towards common interests involves trust and mutual respect with fellow members of the community. Like any group activity, unless everyone works at the common goal, the community will not be successful.

For these reasons, your tutors will give you opportunities to socialize with your fellow students online. You will work in online discussion forums or discussion boards. Some of these discussion boards will be aimed at enabling the students to get to know each other (see Activity 3.1). (For more information about online discussion forums, please see Chapter 6.)

Introducing yourself to your fellow students and tutor in a discussion forum message is a little like meeting people for the first time. First impressions count. You might, however, feel a bit shy and be tempted to just post a brief message saying who you are and where you work and live. Try to be a little brave and include something in your message that gives the reader a taste of who you really are – reveal a little of your personality (see Activity 3.2).

Your tutors may set up a number of other discussion forums that help you to socialize with your fellow students. For example, there may well be an online 'virtual student coffee bar' which is a discussion forum where you will be encouraged to talk about the things that you might in a real coffee bar on a university or college campus: a TV programme, a new film you have seen, a restaurant you visited, a political issue, your holidays.

Once you have begun to generate some discussion with your colleagues, your tutors will begin to set up other forums for you. These will be, by then, much more directed towards the learning outcomes for the course. Salmon (2002: 1) calls these e-tivities and the main features of these discussion items will include:

- some information, stimulus or challenge ('the spark');
- online activity or piece of work, which will involve you and your fellow students making some kind of contribution to a discussion;
- an interactive or participative element, such as responding to the postings of others;
- summary, feedback or critique from your tutor ('the plenary');
- all the instructions you need to take part in the activity ('the invitation').

(Salmon 2002)

Activity 3.1

Introductions

Here is an example of an early message from your tutor in the discussion forum.
    Read the message and then draft a response.

> Hi everyone! Welcome to the course. It is usual when groups are working together online for each member of the group to introduce themselves. Since we do not really know each other at the moment and we are not likely to meet face-to-face, I wondered if we might add a little something to make it a little more interesting. So . . .
>
> Please click on the title of this forum and then 'new thread' and post a message introducing yourself. Tell us who you are and what you do. Then tell us three 'defining' things about yourself that you are willing to share with the group. I have done mine first to give you an example.
>
> When you have done this – please reply to a few other people's messages, asking them questions and offering comments on their 'defining' things.
>
> Julie

Remember that you need to think about how your message presents your 'persona' to your fellow students. Imagine it as the first time you have met them face-to-face and this is your opportunity to give them a flavour of who you are. What will you say?

Activity 3.2

First response

You drop back into the discussion forum, where you have left your message introducing yourself, an hour or two later and discover the following message from a fellow student. Think about how you might respond to Jean's message. If this were a face-to-face conversation what kind of things might you pick up on in her message? What questions might you ask her about in relation to the information she has given you? In what ways might you find some common ground on which to base an online conversation?

Greetings fellow students (and tutor, of course!)

I'm Jean and I'm really pleased to meet you all. Isn't it strange trying to work like this without being able to see people's faces or hear their voices? I'm really looking forward to this course as it will be new and different, but I'm quite daunted by it.

I live with my husband John and two dogs called Ben and Lucy in a small village near the sea. I work in a care home for older people with mental health problems. I had to think hard about three defining things about myself but here goes . . .

1   I have a passion for food . . . both eating and cooking it and I love to eat out. This shows on my waistline, especially now that I am over 40!
2   I love old movies – especially musicals from the 1950s – particularly anything with Doris Day or Jimmy Stewart – sad huh?
3   I hate 'reality' shows on TV – I think they show a sad side of humanity and I can't bear to watch people embarrassing themselves in that way!

I really hope we are all going to get to know each other through this medium as it feels so strange trying to communicate and work with people you have never met!

Jean

Your responses to these 'invitations' are very important. Box 3.1 has an example of a tutor's posting.

Many students say that they find using discussion forums to discuss issues around their practice and the underpinning theory quite liberating. Some

---

Box 3.1

An example of a tutor discussion board posting

The Ashworth family

Kevin Ashworth is 32 years old. His partner, Tracey, is 15 weeks pregnant and is just about to attend the local antenatal clinic for her 'booking'. James is 7 years old and is Tracey's child by another partner. Kevin, a forklift truck driver at the local paper factory, has a brother 3 years younger than himself who has a learning disability. James' teachers have recently asked to see Tracey because James is expressing behavioural problems at school. He is also bed-wetting at home. Tracey is worried about Kevin. She thinks he might be depressed. He certainly seems 'down' and she is not sure why. His mood seems low, he is very lethargic and lacking in energy and he wakes up early in the morning (sometimes as early as 3 or 4 am) and he is unable to get back to sleep. He has had a previous bout of depression – his GP put him on some pills, but he stopped taking them after a week because they didn't seem to make any difference. One of the most worrying signs is that Kevin has lost interest in taking his brother to see his local team play football and he has also lost interest in the darts team of which he is captain.

- What do you think is the likely impact of Kevin's apparent depression on the family? Respond to this question by clicking on the reply button. You can respond to your fellow group members' messages in the same way.
- What else would you want to know about Kevin? For example, would you want to know if he was feeling 'suicidal'?
- In your capacity as a health or social care professional, do you feel that you have a role in supporting people who are depressed?

To help you with this discussion I have placed some information and links in the learning resources section of this site for you to use to consider the issues involved.

Liz

often say that they would not normally feel able to contribute to a discussion in a classroom session as they feel too shy. Downing and Chim (2004) actually recognize this in some research that suggests that people who are normally introverts in classroom settings feel more extravert because they are given time to reflect on what they want to say and they feel less self-conscious. Students also often feel more able to express their views as well as challenge those of other students, especially in relation to attitudes (see Box 3.2). 'Getting along' with other students is quite important in this respect. This does not mean to say that there are not conflicts between learners, but that the important thing is to keep the mutual goal of learning in mind.

The conundrum of time

Time is one thing that everyone is short of in this world today. We live our lives at such a pace that many people feel they are 'time poor'. This is a particular issue for anyone embarking on a course of study. Lewis and Allan (2005) in their research notice that, for many students, time is a key issue and is central to their success in a learning community. The reason it is more important than ever for e-learners is one of e-learning's major advantages – its flexibility. Because of this and the fact that students are not, generally, required to turn up to a certain place, at a certain time on a certain day, there is a danger that students feel they can study at 'any time'. While this is, essentially, true – what it often means is that students do not set aside specific time for their studies and for logging on to make a contribution to the learning

---

Box 3.2

An example of a student discussion forum posting

This is a message from a student following her first online activity:

> I wasn't sure what to expect from this course and I thought I might find it difficult. I wondered if I might prefer to have a proper lecture and would learn less from this approach. However, I take that back now, because I enjoyed it more than I thought I would. I feel I learnt more doing this sort of thing than sitting in a lecture room. I get more involved this way because I don't like to speak up in lectures. It was nice reading everyone else's views and opinions as people came up with things that I hadn't thought about – so thanks everyone. Hopefully I will find future discussion as interesting and beneficial.

> Lisa [not her real name]

community. Consequently, it becomes all too easy to let other aspects of daily life take priority and the e-learning tasks never get done. In this way it is very easy to get behind with weekly e-learning activities and lose touch with the discussions that are taking place. Once you get a little behind, then becoming a lot behind is more likely and it is for this reason that some students fail to complete e-learning courses. This is why commitment is so important. Our advice to you on this matter is as follows:

- Be realistic about the amount of your time the course will take up.
- Make realistic allowances in your life to devote this time to your study.
- Set aside regular time each week for your studies and for contributing to the online learning community.
- Choose a time of day when you are likely to be best able to learn.
- Make this time commitment for a number of shorter periods rather than once a week so that you do not feel daunted when you have not logged in for a week or more.
- If you feel daunted by the amount of discussion you have to catch up on, focus on one or two discussion forums – either the most recent ones or the one that most interests you.
- Do not beat yourself up if you think you are not perfect and do not give up if you think you are getting behind.
- Use the tutor – these individuals will be skilled at supporting you in the e-learning environment and will be very keen to help you out if you are struggling – they will probably have guessed and may contact you to see if you are OK anyway. It is best to contact them before they contact you!
- Try to have some fun in the discussion forums – socializing with other students is thought to be an important part of learning.
- Try not to become a **lurker** who reads discussion postings but does not participate – you will enjoy your learning less and not feel you are part of the community of learners.
- Focus on any assignment you might need to do right from the beginning.
- Give yourself treats for the work you have done!

Information exchange

Traditional methods of learning, such as lectures, are perceived by many as passive modes of learning (Foreman et al. 2002). Students are perceived as empty data storage systems waiting to be filled with exciting and useful data by direct download from the 'teacher'. This is rarely the case as students bring much to the learning situation. Most teachers recognize this and incorporate aspects of students' prior knowledge and interaction into their teaching methods. E-learning (and, indeed, other forms of distance and open learning) takes a different approach. You need to begin to view the tutor as the facilitator of learning rather than a font of knowledge. Tutors rarely know everything about a given subject area – what they are really good at, though, is enabling you to identify sources of learning and make the best of them.

You also need to acknowledge that your fellow students have much to teach you. Your tutor will engage you in activities that involve you searching for information for yourself. This way you are sure to find information that is relevant to you. However, it does not end there. You will then be expected and encouraged to share the information you have found with other students. You might, for example, be asked to summarize what you have learnt and discuss the issues raised with other students. This helps you not only to consolidate your own learning but also to enhance that of others.

Even though some of the information and reading materials you need for your learning will be provided for you, you need to work hard at finding the information you need for your learning, especially if your searching and researching skills are still developing. You can learn more about this in Chapter 5. What is important too is that you are willing and able to share and interpret what you find with your fellow students and to discuss the issues it raises in detail so that your learning becomes an active process.

Knowledge construction

When you have gathered information and started to integrate it into the way you think about your learning and practise as a health or social care practitioner, you will have begun to construct meaningful knowledge for your own needs. Once you have begun to do this you will be able to put the ideas and information together as knowledge that is useful specifically to you and applies to your situation. Using online discussion forums where you share your thoughts and ideas on the knowledge you are constructing from your learning is very stimulating. You will develop opinions and ideas that are based on carefully considered information and debate their implications with fellow students.

Development

Learning is student directed. Learning opportunities are facilitated by the e-tutor, but responsibility for accepting these opportunities and taking responsibility for what is learnt is taken by the student. Once you have made sense of your learning materials you will be able to apply what you have learnt to specific situations in your everyday life and in your practice. This makes the role of the learner a very active one. You will use the knowledge you have gained to develop your learning in the future.

Support, mentoring, supervision and buddies

E-learners can often feel isolated by the lack of face-to-face contact. After all we are all used to working and living in a world where contact with others is the norm and part of the culture in which we live. However, e-learning does not expect that you should cope with everything on your own. Aside from your e-tutor and fellow students, there are a number of other relationships you can develop. One or more of the following can be very helpful in providing you with support and advice:

- a mentor
- a supervisor
- a buddy.

A mentor

A mentor is an individual you select (or sometimes is selected for you) who has some knowledge and experience that may be useful to you and is willing to share it in the course of your learning. These individuals can often be people with whom you work or who have an understanding of the culture of your work and use this to help you facilitate your learning. They use their experience to support you where you are less experienced. Your mentor should be someone for whom you have respect in relation to your area of study. You can negotiate a level of support from them and seek their assistance on a regular basis. Their role is purely supportive and they should not be threatening to you. Selecting a mentor who has experience of online learning or of some of the technology you will be using can be very helpful as they are likely to be able to help you out with minor technical problems. Your mentor should be able to provide you with support for many aspects of your learning and be able to answer questions about the issues raised in the subject area you are studying as well as issues around study itself.

A supervisor

A supervisor is someone with whom you have a much more formal relationship. This individual is most likely to have some role in overseeing your ability and competence in the workplace. Even so, they can be very good at providing you with constructive feedback on your progress. It is important that your supervisor has both an understanding of your needs as an e-learner and is able to support you in your learning exploits.

A buddy

A buddy is a much more informal term. It is used to signify a work partner who provides support either in your learning situation or your workplace. Finding a buddy, for example, who has good computer skills can be quite helpful if you need assistance with these issues.

Conclusion

E-learning offers a complete change of focus for learning. The focus is on you, the student, rather than the tutor being centre-stage (Forman et al. 2002). This frees you to learn what you want and/or need to learn, thus making your learning relevant and personal. To engage with this, you need to think carefully about how you approach the learning opportunities offered you. You need to think about your motivation and the time you are able to devote to your studies. You also need to consider your commitment to the other students and your tutor, especially in your participation in online activities and discussion.

References

Downing, K. and Chim, T.M. (2004) Reflectors as online extraverts? *Educational Studies* 30 (3): 265–276.

Forman, D., Nyatanga, L. and Rich, T. (2002) E-learning and educational diversity. *Nurse Education Today* 22 (1): 76–82.

Lewis, D. and Allan, B. (2005) *Virtual Learning Communities: A Guide for Practitioners*. Buckingham: Open University Press.

Salmon, G. (2003) *E-moderating: The Key to Teaching and Learning Online*, 2nd edition. London: Routledge Falmer.

Salmon, G. (2002) *E-tivities: The Key to Active Online Learning*. London: Kogan Page.

Twomey, A. (2004) Web-based teaching in nursing: lessons from the literature. *Nurse Education Today* 24 (6): 452–458.

4 The role of the tutor in online learning

Introduction

This chapter will discuss the facilitation and support you can expect from your tutor in relation to online learning. The aim is to provide you with practical advice on how to gain the most from your tutor in order to enhance your enjoyment of the e-learning experience. Some of the advice and points made within this chapter will also be relevant to tutorial support in any type of learning experience, however, the central theme is online tutorial support.

Teaching and learning

Health and social care education has predominantly moved on from an apprentice-type training to a more adult learning model where the emphasis is on student-led learning, and teachers being facilitators rather than didactic providers of information. This change has been made in order to encourage those undertaking health and social care education to be 'knowledgeable doers' rather than someone who is taught the 'how' but not the 'why' of their role. This involves a shift of responsibility from the teacher to the student and creates what should be a partnership approach to learning. This does not detract from the responsibility of the teacher to provide a programme of study that meets the requirements of the student and the appropriate professional body. It does, however, mean that as a learner you have some responsibility for your own learning. It is for this reason that we have chosen to refer to the online tutor rather than the teacher or lecturer as this indicates better the role in facilitating, guiding and supporting learning.

The content of the programme or module

A major responsibility of the tutor is the curriculum design of the content of any module or programme of study. In health and social care, the overall content and learning outcomes may be determined by the professional body (e.g. the Nursing and Midwifery Council) but there is also generally some discussion between tutor and service providers as to what they perceive is relevant to a particular module or programme. The tutor should be considered as someone who is very knowledgeable in the subject matter but will not generally arbitrarily decide on the content of your study. The tutor will however design the module or programme in terms of making the order of the content logical, and writing aims and learning outcomes. The aims and learning outcomes are important to you as a learner because they tell you what you should get from your study and what you should be able to do when you have completed it.

An e-learning module or programme differs significantly from the more traditional classroom approach in terms of content and design. The tutor cannot easily replicate a lecture online and has to design activities that give you the best opportunity to learn the subject matter and make it meaningful. Health and social care education has to be applied to a range of different practice areas and this can be quite a challenge to curriculum design especially when learning is online. Learning outcomes identify the objective of your learning and signpost where you should be on completion of the module or course. The e-learning process has to be designed to enable you to gain the knowledge and skills identified by the learning outcomes. As a learner, therefore, it is important that you understand that the tutor will have provided you with activities that are relevant to achievement of the outcomes and are not just arbitrary time fillers (see Box 4.1). Activities will be organized in such a way as to structure your learning logically and each one will build on the previous to develop your knowledge.

Support in relation to your technical skills

Online learning requires you to be able to use the system being used to deliver the module or course. While it is true that you have some responsibility not to select an e-learning course if you have no technical computer skills at all, it is also true that there is a need for your tutor to provide a good level of

---

Box 4.1

Learning outcomes and activities: an example

Outcome 1
The learner will be able to describe the physiology of the respiratory system.

Activity
An online quiz relating to respiratory physiology.
   This would allow the tutor to test the full breadth of your knowledge rather than just a single element.

support with using the virtual learning environment. To achieve this, some tutors prefer to offer an induction session that is face-to-face at the institution providing the course. This approach has the added advantage of allowing students and tutors to get to know one another. This type of session will provide you with a demonstration of the system and its component parts and for you to try it under supervision. You can ask questions and clarify expectations at such a session.

However, this is not always possible due to geographical and time constraints. The alternative is for your tutor to provide you with a series of exercises that will take you through the elements of the virtual learning environment in simple steps before you start to use it for learning the content of your course. These exercises are essential for you to familiarize yourself with the learning environment before you are faced with using it to address the subject matter of the course. There may be exercises that seem unnecessarily simple to you, but they are designed to support everyone and are therefore pitched at a very simple level to ensure that everyone gets the best opportunity to gain confidence in using their virtual learning environment. Within this online guidance there will be opportunities for asking questions, just as there would be in a face-to-face session. It is important that you do ask questions, as your tutor will be keen to ensure that any difficulties are resolved quickly and that you do not get frustrated. Your tutor will also value your questions as these will help clarify how you are managing.

The online demonstration will need to be supported by written information. This is because one run through the exercises or a single demonstration may not be enough to ensure that you are proficient in navigating round and using the virtual learning environment. Your tutor should provide a guide to using the system for you to refer to whenever you need. The guide may be provided in hard copy or may be an electronic version within the learning environment. Providing written information does not mean that your tutor will not answer any further questions you might have; you should not be frightened to ask. Your tutor will not want you to struggle on your own and certainly will not want you to lose out on your learning because of a technical problem. An email or a telephone call can often quickly resolve your difficulties.

Course information

Your tutor will provide you with information pertinent to your course. This will include the rules and regulations associated with the institution running the course. You will need to read this information carefully. Many tutors will provide a summary of the main points you need to know but there will be issues you might not anticipate needing to know within the handbook provided by the college or university.

Course information will also include details of marking criteria for your course and referencing instructions. Again your tutor may well provide additional information regarding these important issues.

Socialization

As discussed in Chapter 3, a very important element of successful online learning is the interaction between learners and their tutor as well as with other students. Without the benefit of the contact you would normally get in the classroom, it can be quite difficult sometimes to relate to your fellow learners. The online tutor therefore plays a significant role in encouraging socialization between students.

To start some interaction your tutor will ask you to introduce yourselves online using a specific discussion board for this purpose as described in Chapter 3. The tutor will generally begin the process by providing an example for you to follow.

Each tutor will use a slightly different format but common methods are the provision of a mini-biography (as in Box 4.2) or asking you to tell the group some things about yourself that are personal to you. The tutor will provide you with clear instructions as well as an example. Once the initial responses are posted then the tutor will encourage further discussion; this could possibly

---

Box 4.2

Example of tutor's introduction

Hi Everyone,

Welcome to the Advanced Critical Thinking Skills module: I hope you will all enjoy it.

As you know I am your tutor for this module, I have been a full time nurse teacher for 11 years now and thoroughly enjoy it. My clinical background is midwifery and neonatal care and I started teaching as the tutor for the ENB 405 Special and Intensive Care of the Newborn course. Although I still maintain clinical links with neonatal care I now teach a range of topics and critical thinking is obviously one of these.

I am married and have two dogs, Boddington (after my husband's favourite beer) and Monty. I love walking (fortunately!), reading, cross stitch and photography. I am also a Newcastle United fan.

I am looking forward to hearing all about you.

Liz

be in relation to a theme such as common sporting or other interests. For example, your tutor may ask questions or introduce a piece of news relevant to the theme. You should respond to your tutor's encouragement and follow the lead they are providing.

Encouraging socialization necessarily means that there is some informality in your interaction with your tutor. You may find this difficult, but it is very much a feature of online learning and, indeed, of a more adult learning model. Socializing online will also include some humour and fun and again this is not inappropriate, although you do need to be careful about making 'jokes' that can be easily misunderstood in the online setting. In classroom learning, you would have breaks when you would socialize and discuss things unrelated to the course content and the socialization you experience online is meant to be equivalent to this. Respect for each other is important despite the informality, and you and your tutor should be able to demonstrate mutual respect as well as developing a more informal relationship than may occur with other methods of teaching and learning. This is discussed in more detail in Chapter 9.

Your tutor may use a variety of methods of maintaining the socialization between you and your fellow students throughout your course. These will include discussion board 'coffee shops' and topical discussion threads that are not related to the formal course content. Your tutor can provide the forum for discussion but it is up to you to contribute and to interact with others. Tutors will offer more of themselves online than they perhaps would do in a classroom in order to facilitate socialization and they will expect you to give something in return (see Figure 4.1).

Ground rules

Your tutor will have provided you with the college or university rules and regulations relevant to your study but online learning needs some basic ground rules to ensure that students gain the most from the experience. Your tutor will facilitate agreement of these and may have some rules that they feel necessary for smooth running of the course. Many of the ground rules set that relate to your tutor will be around what you can expect from academic support (discussed below) and how often your tutor will access discussion boards and other relevant sites to provide feedback and facilitate further debate. They should give you an idea of how often and when they will be logging on, so that you have an idea of when the tutor is likely to respond to postings or comment on the emerging discussion. Ground rules will also be set relating to your commitment to studying online. You will be expected to set time aside to work through the learning materials and undertake the activities. Your tutor may feel that reminders are necessary if you fail to contribute to discussions or appear not to be spending enough time on your studies. The ground rules will differ from course to course as these will depend on the content, professional requirements and the learners' ability (Christianson et al. 2002).

Address:	http://..........	
	Courses> Critical Care of the Newborn>Coffee Shop	
	92379: Critical Care of the Newborn	
Course Menu Announcements Course Information Learning Resources Web Links Discussion Boards Chat Room Email Tools Help		**Coffee Shop**
		Monday 25th September 2006
		Since you are all a little shy about using the discussion boards I thought I would introduce a topic which should hold no fears for anyone - food and drink. Tell me what you would like served up in this virtual coffee shop. I would like good quality tea (made in a pot with boiling water) and chocolate éclairs with real diary cream! Liz Now you are talking!! Hot chocolate, toasted tea cake with lots of butter! Cheers everyone Wendy A big breakfast bacon tomato eggs sausages etc cooked to perfection followed by a nice pot of tea. Lynn Top bloke's breakfast, none of your diet food nonsense here!! James

Figure 4.1 Example of a socialization posting

Learning materials

The role of the tutor in any learning experience is to provide teaching relevant to the topic and to the learning environment. Your online tutor will provide a range of resources and materials for you in relation to the subject being studied. Online learning does not, however, mean that you will be provided with a large amount of written material that you simply read. Different approaches will be used depending on the subject but a central concept of e-learning is learning by doing rather than by being spoon fed information. This appeals to some learners (but not all) and will depend on individual learning style. Online tutors do their utmost to vary the teaching strategies they use to ensure that they maintain interest and meet the needs of their students.

It is important that as a learner you undertake the activities and provide the responses asked for. Your tutor will set up a discussion forum to facilitate your responses to the activities set. Just as it is important that you undertake the activities and provide responses, it is also important that the tutor provides you with feedback and discussion in relation to your responses. Your tutor might also summarize the contents of a discussion at the end to ensure that everyone understands what has been said and to make it easier to retain the learning progress made. In order to test your understanding, your tutor may ask questions about the information you have provided. This does not mean you are wrong necessarily; your tutor is testing your knowledge or your ability to support your argument. This questioning should therefore be taken in the spirit it is meant and not regarded as criticism; most tutors will take care to ensure that their intentions are not misinterpreted but this can occur despite their best efforts.

The activities listed in Box 4.3 are some common examples of e-learning activities associated with health and social care. These, and your use of them, will be discussed in more detail in Chapter 7. You may encounter others designed by your tutor as well.

Reading is an important aspect of learning and the higher up the academic ladder you climb, the more reading is expected. Generally, if you are given reading to do, then you will be expected to provide some feedback or undertake some activity associated with the literature. Reading material and then discussing its content and meaning is a good way of helping you to understand what you are reading and to integrate it into your thinking. Your tutor will be encouraging you to read critically and not accept information simply because it is published. Whether reading is provided as a specific activity or as an associated reading list, your tutor will assist you with a selection of appropriate reading, both for the topic and the level of the course. You will also be directed to web-based reading, generally by means of links within your virtual learning environment. Although reading lists will be provided in relation to specific learning activities and an overall indicative reading list will be included in your course information, this is by no means all the reading available. Part of your learning is to find further literature relevant to the subject and your practice (see Figure 4.2).

Box 4.3

Types of learning activities

- reading
- web-related reading
- articles to critically appraise
- quizzes and tests
- scenarios
- problems to solve
- material to apply to your own practice
- discussion and debate about a topic.

Address:	http://..........	
	Courses> Social Policy and Health Care>Learning Materials	
	46742 Social Policy and Health Care	
Course Menu		**Learning Materials**
Announcements		**Monday 2nd October 2006**
Course Information		
Learning Resources		The literature tells us that there is a certain
Web Links		ambiguity about social policy. Using your own
Discussion Boards		knowledge and the definitions above try to come
Chat Room		up with an explanation of what you think social
Email		policy is and post it in the discussion forum.
Tools		
Help		You do not need to be precise. It is helpful for
		you just to have some ideas. Ideas and thoughts
		are a good basis for an interesting, stimulating
		and educational discussion!
		Try to bring this into perspective by thinking
		about how and what social policy impacts on the
		lives of the individuals who are your patients or
		clients.
		You might also want to think about the meaning
		of the term "welfare"

Figure 4.2 Example of a tutor's online activity message

Quizzes and tests may feature within your online learning depending on the nature of the subject matter. Your tutor will choose this method of activity where the subject matter is broad. Examples of where these are useful are in relation to topics such as anatomy and physiology, sociological theory, and technical aspects of care such as electrocardiography. Your tutor will ensure that only the two of you will have access to your score so you will not have to worry about competitiveness.

Scenarios and problem-solving exercises lend themselves to both health and social care and to online learning. The central tenet of health and social care education is to be able to apply knowledge to practice and these activities are useful tools to help you with this. Virtual patients or clients and other formats may be used by your tutor, who will provide you with the background information you need to consider the issues highlighted in the activity. These activities in particular are helpful in reducing the theory/practice gap that students find particularly difficult and the online medium allows you to discuss with your tutor and other learners barriers to applying theory to practice. Your tutor will fully understand that these barriers do exist so do not assume that they will not discuss and debate the issues with you. Your tutor, however, will expect that you will work together to constructively address the problems rather than just accepting they exist. Further information about learning clinical and communication skills online can be found in Chapter 10.

Tutorial support

We have already mentioned that your online tutor will provide feedback on your responses and offer questions or discussion points. This is very much a part of the ongoing support you can expect from your tutor, whose role is to guide and reinforce your learning (see Figure 4.3).

You can access this guidance and support in relation to the course learning material either through the relevant discussion forum to be shared with other learners or by contacting your tutor on an individual basis. You can ask for guidance in respect of any of the activities or the subject matter itself. The tutor will support you with guidance on academic issues such as critical appraisal of literature, terminology or the subject itself. You can also ask for help with applying the theory to practice. You should never feel that you are asking irrelevant or 'silly' questions; it is always better to ask than to keep quiet and not learn a relevant aspect of the material.

In many respects it can be easier to ask for ongoing support online as the tutor is easier to access and the impersonality of electronic communication can sometimes reduce shyness. However it is important to remember that your tutor will not be online all the time and your course will not be their only responsibility. There may well be a time lag before you get a response. The lack of an immediate response to your query can sometimes be off putting but you will have to be patient. Being an online tutor is a demanding role but most tutors do try to access the virtual learning environment regularly and

Address:	http://..........	
	Courses> Social Policy and Health Care>Week 1 Discussion	
	46742 Social Policy and Health Care	
Course Menu		**Week 1 Discussion**
Announcements		**Monday 2nd October 2006**
Course Information		
Learning Resources		Thanks for this Lynn.
Web Links		What do you think is a basic standard of living
Discussion Boards		and why does this have an impact on health and
Chat Room		social care? Liz
Email		
Tools		
Help		

Figure 4.3 Example of a tutor's facilitation message

check their emails on a daily basis at least. Your tutor will probably set ground rules about the time span you can expect in respect of this; each tutor will be different as each will have different workload pressures.

Where 'real time' responses are needed then your tutor can arrange a tutorial session in the chat room. Here you can communicate simultaneously and you can gain clarification for any responses you do not understand or are not sure about. Some tutors will schedule chat room tutorials into the programme of study; others will arrange them by request.

Being an e-learner does not exclude you from accessing the 'normal' means of gaining tutorial support. You can arrange face-to-face tutorials if it is feasible from a distance point of view and telephone calls can be useful if you have questions or need clarification of an issue before you continue with your studying. You will need to remember, however, that your tutor will have other demands on their time and it is wise to make an appointment for telephone and face-to-face tutorials.

Academic support

A vital aspect of a tutor's role, whatever the type of course, is supporting students with their assignment. Generally, in classroom teaching there is an opportunity for the tutor to go through the assessment strategy and criteria with the student group and to conduct assignment workshops. This can be replicated online by ensuring that there is clear, accessible information about the assessment and the criteria that you are required to meet. The information provided will include the 'extra' explanation of the criteria that you would normally get verbally. Assignment workshops can be conducted online by means of the discussion board or using the chat room for a group tutorial. Tutors will answer any questions about the assessment throughout your course so always ask if you are not sure what is expected of you.

The element of academic support that students often find the most useful however is individual support in relation to their assignment. As already stated individual tutorials can be accessed via the chat room for real time communication and your tutor will offer the same guidance here as can be sought at a face-to-face tutorial. Just as with a traditional approach to a tutorial, your tutor will appreciate some preparation on your part. This may be questions you want to ask or a plan of your assignment that you have sent your tutor in advance. It is important to use your tutorial time effectively so this preparation will help you get the most from your tutor.

You may wish to ask your tutor for comments on draft work. Again, just as with more traditional teaching methods, this is a service provided by your online tutor. There will be ground rules about how and when this is done and these will differ from institution to institution. Most tutors will see one draft although some will see only a partial draft. Tutors will make their approach explicit from the outset but if you are not sure it is wise to ask. Feedback can be provided by email or by chat room tutorial. Tutors need time to read and review draft work: it is common to allow a week for this though you may get it back sooner. There are times when tutors have a large amount of draft work to deal with and this will increase the time you have to wait. For this reason some tutors will not see draft work in the final week or so of the course as they feel you will not have time to act appropriately on their feedback. Online tutors, like any other, will not mark your draft and will not tell you whether it will pass or fail. They will provide you with pointers to improve your academic style and the content of your essay but they do not give detailed feedback on what you need to write. Most tutorial feedback consists of a set of questions or suggestions relating to further expansion of your discussion. Do not be disheartened by the amount of feedback you receive – it might mean your work is poor but it may also mean it is not; remember that if you receive a mark of 60 per cent on a piece of work there is still 40 per cent that could be substantially improved! Tutorial advice is designed to help you both to succeed with your assignment and to improve your overall academic writing skills; it is therefore well worth accessing and acting on. Should you be unfortunate and need to resubmit your assignment, your online tutor will provide you with constructive feedback in relation to what you need to do to improve your work sufficiently to pass.

Support for practice-based learning

Although possibly based at a distance from you, your online tutor can support your learning in practice. This can be achieved by

- giving clear guidance on the practice requirements
- answering queries
- providing online materials and activities relevant to practice
- offering guidance for mentors.

Chapter 10 discusses online learning and clinical skills in more detail; however, where practice is an aspect of the course your online tutor will support this.

Pastoral support

Supporting students with issues that impact on their learning experience is very much a part of university life. Online students do not need to miss out on this. Your online tutor will be able to provide support and guidance in relation to personal problems that occur during your studies and which affect your ability to manage your time effectively. Your tutor will be able to advise you about whether you may be able to have extra time to submit your assessed work or direct you to other services within the institution which may be able to help. This can be achieved by one-to-one communication over the telephone or by email to ensure your confidentiality is maintained. It should be made clear however that pastoral support is not, and does not include, counselling (Howatson-Jones 2004).

Part of the pastoral support offered may be in relation to your further personal development. Your tutor can offer advice about what other academic courses are available or what activities might be useful to consolidate your learning. Advice may be available in respect of putting together your evidence of professional development for your professional body where this is required.

Disability support

Having a disability is no longer a bar to gaining continuing education. Within health and social care there are roles that cannot be performed with certain types of disability but there is also a growing recognition that flexibility and ingenuity can facilitate wider access. Disability need not necessarily exclude students from an online course. Indeed the Special Educational Needs amendment to the Special Educational Needs and Disability Act 2001 clearly states that disability needs must be anticipated and that course design should not disadvantage individuals. Software can be used to assist with visual impairment and for those with mobility problems an online course can be a useful means of gaining professional development as it reduces travelling. Support and advice can be obtained from your online tutor, who can ensure that you are introduced to the appropriate services to help with your studies.

An increasingly common problem, largely because of improved under-standing, is dyslexia. Tutorial support and advice can be obtained from your online tutor, who can also gain guidance from colleagues with experience in helping students with dyslexia and similar types of disability.

If you have any type of disability which may adversely affect your learning experience, you do need to let your tutor know. They cannot help if they are not aware but if they do know there is often a considerable amount of assistance they can offer or direct you to.

Conclusion

Online tutors can provide a wide range of support and assistance to learners. The online tutor is committed to providing students with high quality professional development that is tailored to their needs both from a professional and personal perspective. Support with academic and pastoral issues is as much a feature of e-learning as it is in traditional approaches to teaching. It is important to remember, however, that the role of the tutor in online learning is very different from that of other learning methods. It is much more facilitative and you must expect to be offered opportunities for learning rather than being spoon fed with information.

Ground rules will be set with regard to access and the timing of responses but students can find that the flexibility of online support gives them better access to their tutor than classroom-based courses. Support is certainly equal to what you would experience in a traditional learning environment.

References

Christianson, L., Tiene, D. and Luft, P. (2002) Web-based teaching in undergraduate nursing programs. *Nurse Educator* 27 (6): 276–282.
Howatson-Jones, L. (2004) Designing web-based education courses for nurses. *Nursing Standard* 19 (11): 41–44.

5   Using online study resources

Introduction

Central to health and social care study is the use of online line study resources such as **electronic databases** and **search engines**. This is increasingly important in e-learning as electronic access to reading and learning materials means that there is less need to visit libraries and receive large documents by post. In this chapter, you will be given practical advice on how to use online resources successfully and some exercises will be provided to help you with this. This will include advice on how to assess the value of websites and other material. Central to this will also be a discussion of the role of evidence-based practice and how online learning can be linked to outcomes in practice through this agenda.

A number of web/Internet-based resources will be discussed in this chapter. The majority of these are based in the United Kingdom or United States. These should, however, be accessible by many readers across the globe and will give non-UK/US based readers an overview of what is likely to be available in their own country.

The social life of information

The recent period in global history – from the 1980s onwards – has often been dubbed the Information Age. This relates to the fact that information now moves faster than physical travel as a result of innovations such as the telephone, the personal computer and the Internet. Information technology is a term used to identify the process that enhances the speed and efficiency of the transfer of information.

In the twenty-first century, we are bombarded with opportunities for information and many individuals now head straight for the Internet whenever they want to know something. There are some pitfalls with this approach to life and this is put very well by Brown and Duguid (2000) in their book, *The Social Life of Information*:

> Living in the Information Age can occasionally feel like being driven by someone with tunnel vision. This unfortunate disability cuts off the

peripheral visual field, allowing sufferers to see where they want to go, but little besides. For drivers, this full attention to the straight ahead may seem impressively direct. For passengers who can see what the driver does not it makes for a worrisome journey.

(Brown and Duguid 2000: 1)

The world is now awash with information and finding your way through the complicated channels to the right piece of information for you can be fraught with dead ends and non-starters as well as a huge amount of information to reject before you reach what you need. This chapter hopes to help you find your way through the mass of information available to you via an Internet connection. Fortunately, if you know where to find them, there are now many very helpful ways of accessing the information you want and avoiding a mass of material that is useless or irrelevant to you. What you want to do is to find appropriate reading material with which to support your learning and to back up the things you want to say in your written work. This chapter doesn't have the scope to tell you about all the sources you will find helpful, but it aims to make sure you know about the most useful ones for students of health and social care.

First port of call

In an age when information is considered to be so freely available it is often easy to miss some of the more obvious options. To this end, we recommend that you go, first, to three places:

- your course handbooks and guides
- the websites for your course, department and university or college
- the virtual learning environment that supports your course.

Your course and module handbooks and guides (either **hard copies** or digital versions) have been designed by your tutors to provide you with written advice about your learning. To this end they will provide reading lists and lists of websites that relate directly to the things that you need to learn for specific aspects of your course. We strongly advise you to spend some time becoming familiar with your course handbooks and guides so that you are conversant with the information they contain. For example, course handbooks often contain extremely useful reading lists, which students unfortunately often ignore. Such resources, specifically selected by your tutors, can be invaluable in kick-starting your knowledge and understanding of the subject matter.

Equally, the websites and VLE for your course or module will contain a great deal of very pertinent information. Having a good knowledge of what is there and keeping an eye on any new additions can save you quite a lot of time. Your tutors will have provided a host of downloadable reading matter as well as links to appropriate websites that you will find invaluable in your learning.

The library

As a student at a specific institution you will, of course, have access to the facilities available in the library at the university or college that is providing your course. Many health and social care providers often have some form of library facilities for their staff. If you are studying from some distance, visiting a library may not be an economical option for you in terms of either time or financial resources. However, if the library is near enough for you to visit it, there are a number of advantages in doing so:

- You will have the opportunity to browse along shelves of books, picking things up and putting them down. The sights and smells of a real library can be very motivation enhancing and you feel like a 'proper student'. This experience, we hope, will never be replaced by the computer revolution.
- Books are often a useful way to get an overview of a particular subject area. In many ways, they are not as useful as journal articles as the information contained in books is less likely to be up to date. However, books often contain the information you need to understand the subject area enough to be able to calculate what other information you are looking for.
- There is access to all manner of help within a library. Most university and college libraries are well endowed with computers that are networked and Internet connected so that you can search for information about resources you need for your studies. However, the best aspect of a 'real' library (as opposed to a 'digital' one) is that library staff will be available to help you with your search for information, whichever way you want to do it.

Most libraries now have some kind of online catalogue that will allow you to search for material and enable you to ascertain if a trip to the library is worthwhile. If the library is at some distance from you it may well be worth considering taking a whole day to pay a visit so that you need to do so only the once. Before you set off you need, however, to make sure you know exactly what you are looking for and where in the library you might find it. This will save time and make your trip worthwhile. Visiting the online catalogue to check what is available will help immensely in ensuring you avoid aimlessness once you get there.

It is worth remembering that some education institutions will often send books out to students that are studying at a distance, so check with your library if such a service is available. Some professional organizations, for example, the Royal College of Nursing, also provide library services to their members (www.rcn.org.uk). Also, don't forget your local public lending library, as this may well be an additional, and more local, source of information. Many health and social care courses involve studying local populations in relation to their health and social care needs.

National libraries such as the British Library (www.bl.uk) house massive amounts of written material and offer a number of online services to professionals, students and researchers.

Some texts are now available as electronic or e-books. Your library should be able to give you a list of which are available and how to download them.

Electronic study resources

Before the 1990s, most students of health and social care had very cumbersome and time-consuming ways of finding literature about the subjects they wanted to study. On the whole, it involved a trip to the relevant library and long searches by hand thorough volumes of references to journal articles. The computerization of journals, in particular, has revolutionized this process. In addition to printed texts and reference works, many libraries will now provide access to resources such as journals, books, indexes, government publications, encyclopedias, dictionaries and newspapers in electronic format via the library web pages or some other online route. Often these resources are referred to as **e-journals, e-books, gateways/portals** or databases. Very early on in your course, you should acquaint yourself with the best way to access these resources as it is likely to save you a great deal of time when you need to access study materials, especially for assessed work.

Most university libraries, for example, will also provide a good deal of information about using the electronic resources on their website. Becoming familiar with these is a good way to make sure that you are making the best of these facilities (see Activity 5.1). Some will even contain interactive online tutorials; try, for example, 'InfoVoyager' at the University of Hull, UK found at: http://www.infovoyager.hull.ac.uk/index2.html

Activity 5.1

Online resources

Make a list of the web/online resources that you think are most likely to be of use to you.

Find out the web address for your education institution's library and write it down. You might want to put resources such as this into a **favourites** folder in your web browser.

Passwords

Before we go any further it's important to consider the issue of passwords. In the course of your studies you are likely to collect a good number of user names and passwords that give you personal access to a variety of web-based resources provided by your education institution as well as those you already have from your employer. Keeping track of and remembering passwords can be a challenge, but it remains essential that you keep your passwords safe and private. Never give passwords to anyone else.

If you are based in the United Kingdom, for example, you may find that many online electronic resources are accessible by what is know as an ATHENS user name and password, which can be supplied by your employer or educational institutions. All NHS staff in the United Kingdom are eligible for an NHS ATHENS username. Health and social care workers not working for the NHS may also be eligible and should contact the library for more details. Other public sector workers are able to join this system through an arrangement with their employer and the ATHENS service. The ATHENS system controls access to web-based subscriptions to electronic databases and other resources (see www.athensams.net). It means that, instead of having multiple passwords for a large number of resources, many of them can be accessed with just one password and user name.

Portals and information gateways for health and social care

One of your early ports of call when you are looking for information and learning materials online could be a online portal. A portal is a 'one-stop' website, or gateway, that provides access and links to all kinds of other information sources and gives you easy entry to these kinds of resources. For example, there are two particularly useful ones in health and social care in the United Kingdom: the National Library for Health (NLH) and Social Care Online.

National Library for Health

Formerly the National Electronic Library for Health (NELH), the NLH is just what it says it is, an online resource for access to all kinds of information regarding health and health care. It is an excellent portal for accessing information for health care courses and, indeed, for anyone working in a health care or related settings. The NLH Team (2005) strategy states that:

> NLH will deliver a world class information service, benefiting the NHS by improving the quality of care by enabling evidence based decision-making, and supporting education and research. It will save users' time, extend services to previously unserved groups, and improve the cost

effectiveness of library provision. Services will be delivered to users in a personalised way, electronically and through physical libraries.

(NLH Team 2005: 3)

The site contains access to a large number of electronic resources, giving access to information and journal articles about health and health care. It also provides access to a number of specialist libraries. Access to most of the databases is by an ATHENS password and user name: National Library for Health http://www.library.nhs.uk.

Social Care Online

Social Care Online is an extensive database of social care information. It contains research briefings and reports, government documents, journal articles and website links. The site is updated daily by the site's information managers; access is free. The site is produced by the Social Care Institute for Excellence which is aimed at improving the experience of social care users by promoting knowledge about good practice: Social Care Online http://www. scie-socialcareonline.org.uk. This facility and the NLH provide a formidable resource and are so useful that we recommend that you make the most appropriate one for you the **home page** for your web browser so that they load automatically when you log on to the Internet.

Other websites

A useful resource in Australia is the Joanna Briggs Institute, which was formed to enable a collaborative approach to the evaluation of evidence derived from a diverse range of sources, including experience, expertise and all forms of rigorous research and the translation, transfer and utilization of the 'best available' evidence into health care practice: www.joannabriggs.edu.au/about/home.php#. In the United States there are also a number of sites that are designed to make information easier to find. One example is the Child Welfare Information Gateway: www.childwelfare.gov/pubs/usermanuals/menthlth/index.cfm

In addition to NLH and Social Care Online there are a number of other sites worthy of exploration (see Table 5.1).

Browsing the Web

Sometimes the best place to start a search for information about a specific health and social care topic can be the Internet. This is particularly true if the information you are looking for needs to be very up to date. Providing you are cautious about the value of the information provided by it, the Internet can be a good place to get an overview of a topic area you are studying before you conduct a deeper and more specific search. It can also highlight some of

Table 5.1 Examples of information gateways for health and social care information

Gateway name	Web address	Information
Child Welfare Information Gateway	http://www.child welfare.gov	Formerly the National Clearinghouse on Child Abuse and Neglect Information and the National Adoption Information Clearinghouse, Child Welfare Information Gateway provides access to information and resources to help protect children and strengthen families. A site based in the United States.
Health On the Net (HON)	www.hon.ch	Health On the Net Foundation is an organization promoting and guiding the deployment of useful and reliable online medical and health information, and its appropriate and efficient use. It is a non-profit, non-governmental organization, accredited to the Economic and Social Council of the United Nations
Intute	www.intute.ac.uk	Intute is a free online service providing you with access to the Web resources for education and research. The service is created by a network of UK universities and partners. Subject specialists select and evaluate the websites in our database and write high quality descriptions of the resources. The database contains 113,365 records. With links to both health sciences and social sciences on the front page.
Medical Matrix	www.medmatrix.org	A site containing ranked, peer-reviewed, annotated and regularly updated clinical medical resources.
Ripfa	www.ripfa.org.uk	Research in Practice for Adults (Ripfa) is anewly established research utilization organization for adult social care. Its website contains information designed to assist in care research utilization work in the United Kingdom.
SOSIG (Social-Science Information Gateway)	www.sosig.ac.uk	The service aims to provide a trusted source of selected, high quality Internet information for researchers and practitioners in the social sciences, business and law.

the latest research and government publications and tell you who the 'experts' are.

Searching thorough millions of **web pages** to find the information you are looking for involves using search engines. These are tools through which you can search for Web pages by using key words that appear in many of the documents that are on the Web. Some of the more popular search engines are as follows:

- AltaVista: www.altavista.com
- Ask.com (Teoma): www.ask.com
- Excite: www.excite.com
- Google: www.google.com (there are also various regional versions, such as www.google.co.uk for the UK and www.google.com.au for Australia); it gives you the opportunity to search just within UK Web pages
- HotBot: www.hotbot.com
- YahooSearch: search.yahoo.com

It is often a good idea to use more than one search engine when you are looking for information. Google, for example, is the most popular search engine currently, but it searches only about half of the Web pages available on the Internet and using other search engines will help to widen your search.

The problem with conducting this type of Internet search is that you are likely to accrue such a mass of information that you are unlikely to be able to look at all of it. This can be improved to some degree by being very specific about the search terms you use. You can also use some of the **advanced search** options provided within the search engines to make your search more specific.

Here are some basic tips for searching the web:

- Try to make a plan for what you are looking for. The Internet can be very distracting and will give you many opportunities to get off the track you started on. Try to focus your searches and avoid straying if you can.
- Identify the specific key words that are most likely to be useful in your search – try to think laterally and use words that help to identify the specific aspects of an issue you want to learn about.
- Try to be as specific as possible and include all of the words that might identify the subject area you are interested in. For example, a search of the term 'fall' is likely to come up with a great many websites that refer to Autumn in North America as well as something that happens to humans when they overbalance or trip up. A search for the terms 'falls' and 'elderly' or 'older people' will be more likely to find material that is relevant to your area of interest.
- Try to use search terms that represent the issue in more than your own country or professional field. For example the term 'learning difficulties' commonly used in the United Kingdom is often called 'mental retardation' in the United States.

- When looking for specific material, add words like 'definition', 'article', 'report' or 'book' for example to your search – this will tend to pick up sites and material that are more academic and, therefore, likely to fit your needs (see Activity 5.2). It also helps to remove some of the 'commercial' websites that are aimed at marketing a product.
- When you have found a site it is worth adding it to your 'favourites' list in your web browser so that you can locate it again later (Clarke 2004: 68). You can save these links with names and within folders that will make it much easier for you to find them again when you want to.

Boolean operators

Boolean logic is a simple system for allowing you to combine terms for a search so that you are asking the search engine to look for specific combinations of words. These are useful in all kinds of search engines to enable you to be more specific about what you are looking for and identify materials that are more specific to your needs, thus narrowing your searches

Activity 5.2

Searching the Internet

Using at least two of the search engines listed above, conduct a search for the following.

First search for the term 'e-learning'.
How many **hits** did you get?

Now try searching for
'e-learning health' or 'e-learning social care'.
How many hits now?

Now try
'e-learning health elderly'
or
'e-learning health elderly article'.

Each of these searches should narrow your search down and produce increasingly smaller numbers of hits. There will still be a very large number (probably hundreds of thousands).
   Did you notice much difference between the search engines you used in terms of the links they offered you?

down and helping to avoid less appropriate material. Knowing about them will really help you to make the best of searching the Internet and many other databases.

The three main operators in the system are

- AND
- OR
- AND NOT

These **Boolean operators** are placed between the main words of your search to help the system to know what you are looking for in more detail:

- AND requires all terms searched for to appear in a record.
- OR retrieves records with either term.
- AND NOT excludes terms.

Double inverted commas can be used to sequence operations and group words. Always enclose terms joined by OR with double inverted commas (see Box 5.1).

Internet search engines use Boolean operators differently, so it's important to check to what degree and how they are used in the search engine of your choice before you conduct your search (see Activity 5.3). Boolean operators are also used in electronic database searches for journal articles so please refer back to this section later.

Box 5.1

Example of Boolean operators

Imagine you are trying to find some information on the Internet about homelessness.

If you search for the term "Homelessness", you will find a large number of sites related to homelessness generally.

A search for "homelessness" AND "alcohol" begins to offer you sites that include some articles related to the link between homelessness and alcohol use.

A search for "homelessness" AND "mental health" AND NOT "alcoholism" should make sure that the pages shown are those about homelessness and mental health, but articles that include a discussion of alcoholism have been excluded.

Alternatively if you were looking for both pieces about either "homelessness" OR "refugees", for example, you will find these using the OR operator.

Activity 5.3

Internet search engines

Using an Internet search engine of your choice, undertake a search of the Web for something that interests you. Use a variety of different search terms and use the Boolean operators above with them. Do a number of different searches of the same or similar subject. While you do so make notes about the following things:

- Which search terms worked best for finding information that you wanted?
- How many of the websites on the first two pages of results contained information that was valuable to you?
- How good was the quality of the websites that you found?

Reviewing websites

The Internet, on the whole, is a very 'open' place, by its very nature. Individuals and organizations can post any material they wish on the web (providing it is not illegal). Most of the information on the Internet has, therefore, not been 'reviewed' for accuracy and reliability of content. For this reason you need to be very wary of assuming that all of the material you find on the Internet is reliable and valid information, even though a great deal of it is very useful indeed and may give a you a good start on learning about a specific subject area.

You will find a large amount of material on the web about health and social care. Unless these are electronic versions of articles from peer-reviewed professional journals it is unlikely that they will have been checked for their quality. For this reason you need to think about a number of issues in relation to the material you are looking at. Box 5.2 identifies some of the major issues to consider when assessing the quality of health and social care information on the Internet:

The important thing is to be fully aware that not all information on the Internet is reliable and of good quality and to constantly question the information you are being offered. Remember that your tutors and the educational institution with whom you are studying may well have already provided you with lists of useful websites in a variety of subject areas (see Activity 5.4).

In addition to performing your own general search of the Internet, health and social care workers are fortunate to have access to a variety of gateway sites and other resources giving direct access to relevant information.

Box 5.2

Assessing the quality of information found on the Web

Here are some suggested criteria for assessing the quality of information found in websites relating to health and social care (Edwards 2002; Health On the Net (HON) 2006):

1   **Is it credible?**
    Who has written it or is it anonymous? Do they have authority in this subject? What background and professional standing do the writers have? Has some kind of editorial review process been used to assess the material contained in the site and is it clear how this process has been conducted?

2   **Is it accurate?**
    Is the information complete? Is the information based on sound sources of knowledge such as reliable, good quality research? Do articles contain references to reliable sources of information on the subject? Does the site contain an appropriate disclaimer about inaccuracies in its information? Is all the information justified and dated?

3   **Is the information up to date?**
    Does the site contain information that tells you when the site and/or each piece of information was updated and by whom?

4   **Is the purpose of the site clear and fully disclosed?**
    Is the purpose of the site fully identified? Does the site tell you what the mission of the organization behind the site is? Are all its commercial links and intentions fully disclosed? Is there product advertising within the site? Are sources of funding for the site disclosed?

5   **What links does the site provide?**
    Are the links within the site between related pages useful and reliable? Does the site acknowledge other sources of information and provide links?

6   **Is the site well designed?**
    Is the information on the site fully accessible? Is the information easy to find, access and download? Is the information presented in an attractive and accessible manner?

7   **Does the site encourage interactivity?**
    Does the site provide feedback mechanisms to its authors? Are there facilities for exchange of information between site visitors such as discussion forums?

You can read about these issues in more detail, for example, at the Health On the Net website at: http://www.hon.ch/HONcode/Guide lines/guidelines.html (accessed 24 August 2004).

Activity 5.4

Searching for health and social care information

Using the advice about searching the Internet for information above, conduct a search for sites about an issue that interests you.

Take a look at the quality of some of the sites that appear in your search using some of the criteria above.

What conclusions do you come to about the quality of the information and its usefulness to you?

The Cochrane Library and evidence-based practice

Health care has been striving to achieve an evidence-based approach to practice (Muir-Gray 2000) since the 1970s (Evans 2003) and this has been more recently mirrored in social care (Gilgun 2005). The effectiveness and value of research studies need to be evaluated in order to inform practitioners of the best options in terms of health and social care options (Evans 2003). It would be nearly impossible for each practitioner to keep abreast of all of the research available in their given area of practice, so systematic reviews are conducted to assist with this aim.

The Cochrane Collaboration is an international non-profit-making organization that provides up-to-date, accurate and reliable information about health care interventions, using systematic reviews of the evidence or research available (Chellen 2003: 59). Systematic reviews are rigorously conducted summaries of the research in a given subject area that enable practitioners to consider whether the research is of sufficient quality to be applied to practice.

The Cochrane Library is an online database that contains high-quality, independent evidence to inform health care decision-making. It includes reliable evidence from Cochrane and other systematic reviews, clinical trials and other types of evidence. Cochrane reviews bring the combined results of the world's best health research studies together, and are recognized as the gold standard in evidence-based health care. The Cochrane Library is an excellent source of information for academic work. You can access the entire library free of charge at: www.thecochranelibrary.com.

The library has a number of options for searching for information. There is a basic search window as well as an advanced search option. There is also a **dropdown menu**, giving you the opportunity to look at specific clinical topics. The Cochrane approach tends to focus very much on randomized controlled trials of health care interventions, so the more qualitative aspects of health care tend to be less evident. It is, however, an extremely useful first port of call when you need to access evidence on a particular topic. You will find a wealth of information about how the Cochrane Library works on the site itself.

Online journals in health and social care

Journal (or periodical) articles are the most valued source of information for health and social care studies. They provide information about practice, education and research in a format that is easily designed to be accessible to practitioners.

Your education provider or employer will have purchased access to some of the journals relevant to your subject area on your behalf. These journals will not only be accessible in print or hard copy on the library shelves, but also be available electronically for download from the Internet. There are thousands of journals available in hundreds of subject areas. It is unlikely, therefore, that you will have electronic access to them all. Most universities provide access to those journals considered to be of most relevance to their students and staff within the budget they have available for such resources. Its important to remember that not all information on the net is free of charge (Chellen 2003: 73) – your employer or education provider will have paid for online subscriptions to many journals, but not all of the ones you might perceive as useful. Many of these journals will be accessed from your library website and online catalogue. Often, access to such online resources will be through the use of passwords to ensure that only those authorized to use these resources can do so. Some journals will be accessed via the ATHENS password system, while other journals will have their own passwords for access, which you can obtain from your library staff (see Activity 5.5). However, it is important to remember that not all journals can be accessed in this manner and you may identify a number of articles, which are not part of your institution's subscription. If you feel that such materials are likely to be of considerable use to you, your library may be able to access them for you, possibly at a charge to yourself, or you may be able to download them from the Internet for a charge.

You should be able to conduct a **hand search** of the most recent journals online, as all journals will have online contents pages similar to those found in the print versions of the journals. This hand search approach is a useful way of identifying very recently published material, for example that has not yet made its way into the electronic databases.

Some journals will have online access to articles that are 'in print' but not yet available in a published journal. These articles are those that the publishers have prepared to put in a future or forthcoming journal issue, but that issue has not yet been formally published. This provides access to some of the most up-to-date information available on a given subject and is often the most effective way to access recent research findings. Even so, it is worth remembering, that any research published in journal articles will have been completed at least a year before the article is published due to the length of

Activity 5.5

Electronic journals

Visit your library website and use it to find out which online electronic journals/periodicals are available to you.

Make a list and make notes about how to access each of the journals in your subject area.

time the publication process takes, so it is not as up-to-date as you might imagine.

Using electronic databases to search for journal articles

Finding information in a journal article is probably one of the most important skills a student of health or social care can acquire. Accessing relevant up-to-date information is not only good for your assessed and written work, but also central skills in being an 'evidence-based', 'inquiry-based' or 'research-minded' practitioner. Most health and social care providers and all universities will now provide staff and students with access to a number of relevant electronic databases or indexes (for which a large subscription is often paid by the institution) as well as educational opportunities to allow them to learn about electronic database searching. The secret to being effective in finding articles and other material about the subjects you want to study is to practise using these resources constantly. The art of searching databases is actually relatively simple. If you persevere with using electronic databases you will find it easier and easier to reap the benefits of this approach to literature searching.

There are a number of major providers of electronic databases with which you need to become familiar – the majority of these are related to health care, as this is a burgeoning aspect of health informatics. There are some useful resources for social care too. Table 5.2 provides a list of a selection of databases that will be of interest to you. You will most likely be able to access these facilities via your college, university, portal, VLE or health or social care provider web pages. It is unlikely, however, that you will have access to all of those on the list. Some of the services are provided by a secondary provider. You will need to ensure that you have the correct passwords.

Many of these databases have a variety of features to help make your search easier and more effective including advanced search and limiter facilities. It would be impossible to provide specific guidance on using each of these resources in a textbook such as this. We recommend that you seek assistance from your library or librarian in accessing help and instruction. It is, however,

Table 5.2 Health and social care databases and portals

Provider	Web address (Note: most resources will be accessed via your education provider's systems)	Information
BIDS IBSS	www.bids.ac.uk	Provides access to the International Bibliography of Social Sciences – one of the largest and most comprehensive databases in the social sciences. It indexes over 2,000 periodicals and 7,000 books from 1951 onwards in the core disciplines of economics, sociology, politics and anthropology.
CINAHL – Cumulative Index to Nursing and Allied Health Literature	www.cinahl.com also provided by EBSCOhost	Allows you to trace articles in over 1,200 English language nursing and allied health periodicals plus virtually all publications of the American Nurses' Association and the National League for Nursing. Now includes over 300 electronic journals in full text. American focus.
cancerlit	www.cancer.gov/CancerInformation/cancerliterature	Produced by the US National Cancer Institute, CANCERLIT® is a bibliographic database that contains more than 1.5 million citations and abstracts from over 4,000 different sources including biomedical journals, proceedings, books, reports and doctoral theses.
EBSCO academic search elite	http://search.ebscohost.com	View and print articles in over 1,200 journals from 1990 onwards and find references and abstracts for articles in 1,400 additional journals. Covers journals in the social sciences, arts and humanities, education, psychology, economics, business and general science.
EMBASE	www.embase.com	A biomedical and pharmaceutical database specializing in drug-related topics. It indexes over 3,500 periodicals with coverage extending to 1980. Updated weekly.

JSTOR	www.jstor.org	An electronic journal archive of articles from over 117 electronic journals in fifteen disciplines in the sciences, social sciences and humanities. Coverage extends from the 1880s up to two years ago. Current issues are not included in this resource.
Medline/Pubmed	www.pubmed.com	Provides access to over 12 million MEDLINE citations back to the 1960s, and additional life science journals. It also provides access to many full-text journals, and is expanding to include access to 200 years worth of research from historically significant biomedical journals as part of an ongoing digitization project.
PsychINFO	www.apa.org/psycinfo	Comprehensive indexing and abstracting service in psychology and related fields, covering journals, dissertations and – from 1987 – books and book chapters. Updated weekly.
Synergy	www.blackwell-synergy.com	Provides access to online journals in a variety of subject areas. It holds the content for journals. Enables readers to search for relevant articles, read abstracts for free, print the full text of subscribed-to articles, download citations, and make connections to other relevant research through reference linking.
Web of Science	www.isiknowledge.com	Useful for its coverage of general and multidisciplinary titles, can be used either for looking for articles on particular topics, or as a means of tracing citations – i.e. seeing how a known work or author has been cited (or referenced) by other writers.

worth identifying some of the features of these facilities that are useful for you to know about. Here is a list of the main things you can do with most of the above search engines/resources.

First, you can search for articles using one or a combination of the following example search fields:

- Keyword/s – this search option will identify work that is related to the subject area generally.
- Title word/s – this search option will be much more specific and will search the title of articles looking for the words that you specify.
- Author name – this is useful if you know the name of an author who is an expert or has written a great deal about the field that you are interested in.
- Journal title – this search will enable you to identify articles in specific journals that you know to publish articles in your area of interest.

Second, you can combine the results of two searches by using the 'combine searches' options. For example if you were looking for information about depression following child birth, you could conduct a search for the term 'depression' and another search for the terms 'birth' or 'postnatal'. Combining these searches can make your results much more specific to your needs in the same way that using Boolean operators will do.

Third, a variety of 'delimiters' enable you to search for example by:

- articles published between specific years
- limit results to those in a specific language such as English
- limit to results with links to full text articles
- in some science journals you can also limit your results to issues such as whether animals or humans were the subjects of the article/research.

Once again, practice is the key to successful use of these extremely useful facilities. Setting aside time to explore the facilities you have access to will be time and effort well spent and will enhance your success in finding what you are looking for. It's important to remember that, as with any website, exploring all of the page on your screen and checking to see what happens when you click on certain aspects of the page as there are many excellent options that you will otherwise miss. Also, using the 'Help' sections of the sites is a useful way to enhance your understanding of how to use them.

Once you have a list of articles resulting from your search on your screen, many databases will offer you the opportunity to do some or all of the following:

- Print the list – allowing you to choose the detail you require in the print-out.
- Save the list to a disc to review later.
- Email the list to either yourself or another individual.

Full text links and PDF files

Many electronic databases will now offer a link to the full text of the article either via a PDF file or an HTML file. This means that you do not have to search the online or text journal for the article. However, do not expect this to be the case in more than about 10 per cent of the article references you find in your search at the moment, as this is still a developing facility. You will, most likely, still need to access most articles via the online or printed journal.

Many of the articles and papers that are downloadable from the Internet are made available to you as what is known as a Portable Document Format (PDF file). The creators of the material use a specific kind of software to create the file and offer it to you in a format that is not possible for you to alter in any way – it makes the file easy to access on the web while remaining protected for the publisher. We have provided more detail of this subject in Chapter 2.

Printing reading material

One important aspect of accessing online study materials is printing. You have the option, of course, to read all of the materials you have found to help you study a specific topic on your computer screen. Many students find reading large amounts of text on a computer screen very difficult. Many also like to 'interact' with their reading materials by annotating a printed article with pencil or highlighter pen comments. We would encourage you to take this approach as it assists in gaining an overview of the content of reading material and makes it easier to find what you are looking for when you need to return to the article when completing assessed work for example.

In the case of downloadable materials, however, if you print everything you *think* may be useful, we can almost guarantee that you will only actually read about 10 per cent to 20 per cent of it! Printing materials with paper and ink can be very expensive and eat up a great deal of your study budget. Therefore, we recommend that you take the following approach:

- If you see an article that you think you might want to read and use in your written work save it either to your computer hard drive or other form of portable disc (see Chapter 2) for review later.
- Make sure that your computer or the discs you use have folders and subfolders that make it easy for you to find this material again. Also, make sure that you save the files with names that will allow you to recognize the contents of the article.
- When you have finished searching for materials, review the articles that you have saved to your folders (for example, read the abstract on your computer screen) to see if you still feel that piece of literature meets your needs.
- Print the article off if you still feel it is relevant to your work.

Conclusion

The Internet has revolutionized the way in which we can find learning and reading materials for health and social care. We cannot stress enough the importance of making good use of the online electronic methods of identifying and studying reading materials – time spent working on your skills and practicing them results in enhanced learning and increased success in your written assessments. We recommend, if you are a relative novice or lack confidence in this area, that you return regularly to this chapter and seek help from your tutor, library and educational facilities to make the best of what is available to you.

References

Brown, J.S. and Duguid, P. (2000) *The Social Life of Information*. Boston, MA: Harvard Business School Press.

Chellen, S.S. (2003) *The Essential Guide to the Internet for Health Professionals*, student edition. London: Routledge.

Clarke, A. (2004) *E-learning Skills*. Basingstoke: Palgrave.

Edwards, M.J. (2002) *The Internet for Nurses and Allied Health Professions*, 2nd edition. New York: Springer.

Evans, D. (2003) Hierarchy of evidence: a framework for ranking evidence evaluating health care interventions. *Journal of Clinical Nursing* 12 (1): 77–84.

Gilgun, J.F. (2005) The four corner stones of evidence-based practice in social work. *Research on Social Work Practice* 15 (1): 52–61.

Health On the Net (2006) *HON Code of Conduct for Medical and Health Websites*. Available at http://www.hon.ch/HONcode/Guidelines/guidelines.html

Muir-Gray, J.A. (2001) *Evidence-Based Healthcare: How to Make Health Policy and Management Decisions*, 2nd edition. Edinburgh: Churchill Livingstone.

NLH Team (2005) *National Knowledge Service National Library for Health Strategy 2005–2008*. London: NHS. Available at: http://www.library.nhs.uk/nlhdocs/nlh_strategy_2005_2008v2.doc (accessed 9 August 2006).

Recommended further reading

Chellen, S.S. (2003) *The Essential Guide to the Internet for Health Professionals*, student edition. London: Routledge.

Coe, J.A. (2000) *Computers and Information Technology in Social Work: Education Training and Practice*. New York: Haworth.

Fitzpatrick, J.J. and Montgomery, K.S (2003) *Internet Resources for Nurses*, 2nd edition. New York: Springer.

Kiley, R. (2005) *The Nurse's Internet Handbook: A Guide for Nurses in Primary Care*. London: Royal Society of Medicine.

Menon, G.M. (2002) *Using the Internet as a Research Tool for Social Work and Human Services*. New York: Haworth Press.

6 The virtual learning environment

Introduction

This chapter will provide you with practical advice and tips for working in online learning environments. The practicalities of working in online discussion boards will be the main focus as these are central to the development of e-learning communities and in the learning that follows. The principles of a virtual learning environment remain the same whichever system is used. These principles will be the focus of this chapter, but it will also acknowledge some of the more common systems available to and used within health and social care and higher education institutions in the United Kingdom and elsewhere.

A place to learn

Every student needs a place to learn – a study environment, somewhere to learn, think, discuss and write. Individual and logistic requirements for this environment will vary. It could be argued that, with the availability of mobile technology, it is possible to study just about anywhere in the world and it is true that many people can now, for example, learn while on the move in trains, aeroplanes and cars. In reality, most people have some basic requirements for a suitable physical learning environment. Sufficient space, light and an appropriate temperature tend to be basic requirements. For e-learners, however, the situation becomes a little more complex as a very basic requirement is a connection to the Internet and a computer with all the necessary facilities. For many e-learners, therefore, a computer or a series of computers tends to be the place they consider to be their learning environment.

As discussed in Chapter 3, right from the first foothold of Salmon's (2003) steps to learning, access to computer systems that help students to learn and interact is essential. Without access to these, learning can't take place. Where this computer is sited will depend on the places the student has available. Most students of health and social care will access the Internet from computers at home, at work or on a university campus. It is important to remember, however, that accessibility to the Internet may be in all kinds of other places, ranging from Internet cafés to public libraries and a number of other options.

Having made an Internet connection, students then need to 'go' somewhere to access the study and learning tools and this is most likely to be a computer system known as a virtual learning environment (VLE) provided by the health and social care institution or education institution that is providing the learning support. This is the 'place' where many of the learning activities will happen. It could be argued that the Internet or what is often known as **cyberspace** is not really a place. Human beings tend to take their social cues from their surroundings and, as a consequence, may find the Internet a fairly alien place to be. There are, however, many people who find the degree of interactivity with visual stimuli and with other human beings enriches their material lives. As an e-learner, you will begin to see the place where you connect to the Internet, and the **cyberplaces** where you access learning materials and communicate with your tutor and fellow students, as an interesting and valuable place to be, providing you interact with it in a way that suits your personality and learning style.

A VLE is a computer system that allows learning to take place online via an Internet connection. They are web-based systems and normally can be accessed (with a password and user name) from any Internet-connected computer in the world. This, of course, is central to learning online as it provides the 'place' where students go to learn and meet up with other students and tutors. VLEs enable anyone with an Internet connection to access online learning 24 hours a day, seven days a week. This enables them to make use of the two biggest advantages of learning online because the barriers of physical travel and time constraints are removed to a large degree. With the increase in availability of wireless network connections to the Internet, many students of the future will be learning from their own laptop computers in public places such as cafés, parks and even on beaches – anywhere they choose. It's important to remember, however, that there are some locations that are more conducive to studying than others!

Other names synonymous with this kind of system are:

- **Managed Learning Environment**
- Learning Content Management System
- Learning Support System
- Course Management System
- Virtual Campus
- Community/Learning Portal/Platform
- Online Learning Environment
- Web-based Learning Environment.

A VLE is a set of teaching and learning tools designed to enhance a student's learning experience by including computers and the Internet in the learning process. In very simple terms a VLE allows your tutors and others who work with them to create web pages with which to share information and communication with you without the need for expertise in web design. In turn, the idea is also that the material and tools provided in the VLE are easily accessible and simple for students to use. If you can log on to the Internet, find a website and interact with that site in some way, such as finding information or making an online purchase, you are already most of the way there. The principal components of a VLE package include the following:

- Methods for delivering learning materials online. This will include electronic documents in a variety of forms such as MS Word, MS PowerPoint®, PDF (Portable Document Format), MS Excel and, often, digital images, sound, video and audio materials.
- Access to course documents, such as timetables, handbooks and guides.
- Access to discussion boards/forums/groups where students and tutors can undertake socialization and discussion activities.
- Access to email systems for sending emails. Generally emails are sent to the same email address that the student would use for other purposes rather than setting up a separate address.
- Access to tools that allow the student to change their password and personal details within the system.
- An announcements page that allows tutors to let their students know what is happening (see Figure 6.1).

Address:	http://..........	
	Courses > Working with users and carers > announcements	
	479361: Working with Users and Carers	
Course Menu	**Announcements**	
Announcements	**Fri December 17 2006**	
Course Information		
Learning Resources	Hello Everyone. Welcome to the site for Working	
Books	with Users and Carers. The module team hope	
Web Links	you will enjoy the module. The amount of	
Discussion Boards	information on this site will increase weekly so it	
Groups	is important that you log on at least twice a week.	
Email	I will be posting regular online activities with	
Chat Rooms	which to direct your learning. The first of these is	
Student Tools	already in the discussion board area (just click on	
Staff Contact	the Discussion board button to the left). There are	
Help	a number of discussion forums there, including	
	the opportunity for you to introduce yourselves.	
	If you have any problems don't hesitate to email	
	or phone me. Best wishes. Julie (Module Leader).	

Figure 6.1 A diagrammatic representation of a typical home page for a course-site in a virtual learning environment

Source: adapted from Simpson 2002: 103

The majority of universities and colleges now use VLEs both as a tool for e-learning and to support more traditional modes of learning based on the campus. As e-learners, however, you just can't survive without it and it is really important that you get to know the VLE you are working with really well – it is central in your ability to learn effectively. There are many VLEs commercially available on the market today and your university or college may use any one of them. The important thing to remember is that they will tend to have much the same function as each other but be presented in different ways and styles. Common names for VLEs that you might hear are:

- Angel
- Blackboard
- Bodington
- Desire2Learn
- Dokeos
- Edumate
- Fle3
- LON-CAPA
- .LRN
- Moodle
- Sakai Project
- WebCT.

The above list is purely to give you an idea of some of the names you might hear. This is a non-static, dynamic world, prone to new developments and mergers, so it is difficult to give a definitive list.

It isn't really necessary for students to know much about how these systems work, what's important is that you are able to operate the 'front end/user end' of the system that your course/institution uses. There are many computer software systems that allow all of this to take place. At the beginning of your course you should, as a minimum, receive some instructions about how to access the system, including a set of passwords, and some basic information about using the system. Many education institutions will also have a manual for students to use to get them started on these systems. It is vital that you have access to the VLE as soon as the course starts. If you have any problems getting access, you must make contact with your course tutor immediately and ask for help. Even, if they are unable to help immediately, they will know exactly how to deal with your problem and will solve it as quickly as possible because they will be well aware of the disadvantages to you of not being able to join the online community immediately. If you don't make contact with the tutor, they will probably make contact with you fairly quickly, but it is much better for you to be proactive in seeking help when you need it. The tutor will be well aware that not all students are confident in using these systems and will be really keen to give you a helping hand.

An important aspect of using a VLE is the downloading and use of study materials and guidance made available by tutors. These issues were discussed more thoroughly in Chapter 2. This chapter will, mainly, consider the issues around online communication. Similarly the focus will be on discussion forums and chat rooms, because email has also been dealt with comprehensively in Chapter 2.

One important issue is that of **pop-ups**. Pop-ups are small windows that appear in the foreground of your computer screen while you are browsing the Internet. Pop-ups are often used to display advertising or unwanted content on the screen. They can be integrated into some websites for practical purposes, however. Many VLEs use pop-ups within the system to allow tools to be used at the same time as something else in the background. You can disable pop-ups (which can be quite annoying) but you may find that some features of your VLE will then not work. In order to enable pop-ups, you will need to reset any **pop-up blocker** in your web browser. Most pop-up blocker features work in similar ways and the following is the usual process for re-enabling your pop-ups:

1   Select the Tools menu from the toolbar in your web browser.
2   Choose the 'Turn Off Pop-up Blocker' from the pop-up blocker **submenu**.

Virtual communication tools

Lewis and Allan (2005) describe two main types of virtual communication tools, asynchronous and synchronous tools, and these enable different types of contact between members of the online community and facilitator.

Asynchronous tools

Asynchronous tools enable people to communicate at a time that suits them. Individuals post a message that is held by the system. This message can be read and responded to as and when the recipient comes online. Asynchronous communications take place over time rather than at the same time. Examples of asynchronous tools commonly used in virtual learning communities include email, bulletin/discussion boards/forums and mailing lists. Some examples of discussion forums are shown in Figures 6.2 and 6.3. In this book we will refer to this kind of tool as a discussion board or forum.

Synchronous tools

Synchronous tools enable people to communicate when they log on to the system at the same time; that is they are immediate and live communications. Unlike face-to-face communications, a transcript, archive or record of the communication process is provided by many synchronous tools. Examples of synchronous tools commonly used by virtual learning communities include conference or chat rooms, instant messaging, **Internet telephony** and **video conferencing** (Lewis and Allan 2005: 36.). In this book we will refer to this kind of tool as a chat room. You will find an example of a chat room in Figure 6.4 (p. 94).

Working in discussion boards

In our view, the most important part of the VLE is the discussion board or forum (see Box 6.1). This is what sets e-learning apart from other forms of

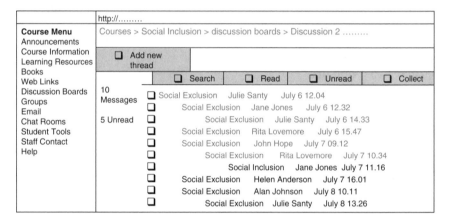

Figure 6.2 A diagrammatic representation of a typical discussion forum in a virtual learning environment

Course Menu	http://.....
Announcements	Courses > Social Inclusion > discussion boards > Discussion 2 ....
Course Information	
Learning Resources	Reply
Books	
Web Links	Hi folks. For this activity you will need to refer to the information sheet
Discussion Boards	you were given with the family profiles. You'll find this in the Learning
Groups	Resources area. In this discussion forum, you will then need to set up
Email	threads for each family and in each one discuss your answers and
Chat Rooms	information gathered too for the questions that were set for you.
Student Tools	• What are the potential social inclusion/exclusion issues of these groups?
Staff Contact	• How can their social inclusion needs be met and by whom?
Help	• What are the professional and inter agency social inclusion issues associated with these groups?
	• How can social inclusion be promoted within these groups?

Figure 6.3 A schematic representation of a typical tutor discussion forum message in a virtual learning environment

distance learning as it allows interaction among students and with the tutor. Asynchronous discussion forums are more flexible than synchronous chat rooms as the participants can log in at any time rather than having to be online at a specific time.

Sit and colleagues (2005) studied student experiences of online learning and found that the students felt that there was inadequate opportunity for

---

Box 6.1

Discussion boards

Discussion boards can be simply explained by likening them to a room with a message board in the following manner:

- A tutor enters an empty virtual room and leaves a message for the students on a board in the room. It asks them to conduct some activity and then undertake some kind of discussion related to some questions identified in the tutor's message.
- Then, one by one, the students will pop in and out of the room to pick up the message from the tutor. But they never actually meet the tutor or each other.
- Some time later a student who has completed the activity drops into the room and leaves a message underneath that of the tutor's, giving a view on the questions posed by the tutor. The student then leaves the room.
- A little while later another student enters the room. This student reads the message from the first student and responds to both this and the tutor's message by writing a message and leaving it on the board just below the first student's messages.
- Other students gradually enter the room to leave their own messages in response to the tutor's message and those of other students.
- Gradually, in this way, a conversation develops over a period of time and the students continue to drop by and leave further messages and responses as the discussion develops.
- The tutor pops in regularly to respond to specific issues and keep the discussion on the right track by leaving encouraging messages and summarizing what is being said.
- At the end of the discussion the tutor returns to the room and leaves a message that summarizes what has been said in the discussion and tells the students that is time to move on to the next discussion or activity.

human interaction to establish peer support and develop in-depth discussion. For these reasons it is vital that each student in the group participates fully in developing online relationships with their peers and tutors.

Often discussion forums will work in the following way:

1   The tutor leaves an electronic message for all students asking them to undertake some learning activity, giving full instructions – this is sometimes called an e-tivity (Salmon 2003). Often this task will involve searching for some specific kind of information and reporting back or some reading in preparation for a discussion of the issues. This message can be known as a **new thread** in that it is the first message at the beginning of a new discussion topic.
2   Each student logs on to the discussion forum and reads the tutor's message. They then undertake whatever task the tutor has asked them to do.
3   One by one the students will return to the discussion board. The first student to return may well set up another new thread, thus starting a discussion about a particular aspect of the learning activity or in response to one or more of the questions or topics set by the tutor.
4   Students will also respond directly to the messages of the tutor and to other students by clicking on the reply button for some or all of the messages.
5   During the development of the discussion the tutor will log on regularly (sometimes at specified times) to make sure that the discussion stays on track, offer advice and assistance and facilitate the discussion by asking questions and summarizing the issues.
6   As the discussion develops an **archive** of the conversation will build up, so that the discussion is there for future reference.

You can see from Figure 6.2 that messages appear indented from each other. This helps the reader to know which message is a response to which. In addition, most systems tend to provide some means of identifying which message you have already read and which you have not. For example, messages that have not been read will be highlighted in some way or will have a little flag next to them. To read the messages, you click on the title of the message.

Here are some tips for working in online discussion forums/boards:

1   Always start a new thread when you are changing the subject and give the thread a name that will make it clear what that discussion is about.
2   When writing a message, begin it with some kind of greeting that allows the reader to know who your message is aimed at. If it is aimed at everyone in the group, for example, you might begin, 'Hi everyone . . .' – or if you want to respond to a specific group member you might begin, 'Hi, Jim . . .'. This helps to make it feel much more like a conversation and makes it clearer where the stimulus for your message comes from.

3 Try to log in at least two or three times a week to pick up and respond to messages. This way, you will keep up with the conversation and not feel overwhelmed.

4 You are not obliged to respond to every message – this would make the discussion boards become busy and uninteresting very quickly, as well as difficult to manage. However, it's a good idea to ensure you do participate in the conversation on a regular basis. This is really no different from having a face-to-face conversation – if you don't join in (this is known as 'lurking' in the e-learning world) – others might assume that you aren't interested and your tutor will be asking if you are still out there!

5 Keep your postings/messages as short as you can. No one wants to read a long-winded diatribe, so it's important to be concise and accurate in what you say.

6 Try to take an equal part in anything your group are asked to do in the way of activities and preparation for group discussions – it will really stand out if you aren't able to contribute because you haven't done the background work.

7 Don't forget that what you say will be there for everyone to read and will remain for some weeks or months to come. You need to be sure that what you are saying is what you want to say. At the same time, you need to try to be natural and not be put off by the fact that you will be able to 're-read' stuff you wrote later.

8 Be as polite as you can and follow the rules of **netiquette** – for example, don't use capital/upper-case letters if you can avoid it – it's the online equivalent of SHOUTING!

9 It's important to be 'critical'. This doesn't mean picking an argument with everyone but it does mean that you don't have to agree with everything everyone says, and you are encouraged to develop an opinion based on your own ideas and research. Be polite but don't just pay lip-service to the discussion. You will learn more if you don't take everything at face-value.

10 If you have taken a break and not managed to log in for a while, say a few days or a week or so, when you return to the discussion board it can feel overwhelming as there will have been a good amount of discussion taking place while you have been absent. The best approach is to start with the most recent discussion forum so that you are joining a 'conversation' that is current. Begin your first message with an apology for your absence and tell everyone where you have been.

11 If you refer to any reading from a website or other source, try to give a reference for it in your message so that other students can find it too.

12 It's a good idea to open a word processor document in a separate window and write your text in that, particularly when you are writing a long posting. When your posting is complete, you can then **copy and paste** the text from the document into the discussion board window. This way you

can use the word processor spell-checker and, if you have saved the file, there is less chance of losing all your hard work if your computer crashes.

13   Try to use the 'social' discussion areas the tutor sets up for you as much as possible – areas such as 'coffee bars' and 'introductions' forums. These will help you to get to know your fellow students and have fun while you learn.

14   Try to play by the rules of normal conversation:

- Be courteous and sensitive and try not to upset your fellow group members.
- Be as honest as you can, bearing in mind the above.
- Think about how you display your attitude towards others and towards issues in the discussion – avoid stereotyping and discriminatory comments.
- Use appropriate language that others will understand.
- Try not to dominate the conversation – give others the opportunity to contribute, especially those who are 'quieter'.
- Be careful how you use 'humour' and 'joking'. It can be easily misunderstood without facial expressions as cues and you are likely to upset other members of the group if your joke is inappropriate.
- Value the views of others and give 'positive' feedback when you can.
- Comment on others' views so that they know you are 'listening' to what they are saying.

Kennedy (2005) says that discussion boards are one of the most productive tools for online learning and that their strength is allowing for reflection, the display of evidence to support ideas, close analysis and critical appraisal of propositions – all very important activities in any student's academic development. Students often tell us that they feel more able to contribute to discussion forums taking place online than they would do in the classroom. This is because they feel they are able to prepare their response and are less likely to be shy online than face-to-face. Some researchers have found that the time given for reflection and the opportunity to engage in discussion allows students who would normally be less active in a classroom-based discussion to behave in a more 'extroverted' way (Downing and Chim 2004), although this will vary according to the students' personality traits and to some cultural cues and norms, and some people may well feel the opposite of this (see Activity 6.1). Working with others in discussion forums can be immense fun. Some people even describe it as 'addictive' when they first start out. You need to make sure that you keep a balance between an appropriate amount of discussion board activity and not allowing it to take over your life!

Working in chat rooms

Chat rooms are facilities that allow you to communicate with one or more people through 'text' messages in real time. These synchronous chats are a

Activity 6.1

A discussion board

You log onto a discussion board for a group in which you have been working for a few weeks and discover the following message from one of your fellow students:

> Hi everyone. I think I'm getting a bit fed up with this e-learning lark now. The tutor doesn't seem to do very much other than tell you what to do and then just comments on what you say all the time. There are some members of the group who aren't really contributing and I think this is really rude and not conducive to successful group working. I think I am about ready to give up on this lark as I think it's a waste of time and I am not really learning anything.

Imagine that the tutor does not see this message for an hour or so after you have spotted it. You feel duty bound to respond. What would you say in response? Do you think this is the right attitude? Do you think that it is important that all students respond to the discussion boards? Think about how this compares with classroom situations. Is e-learning different in terms of what you expect of your fellow students?

useful way to have real time conversations when this is possible or feasible and they can be quite good fun (Clarke 2004). These are less flexible than discussion boards because all of the participants need to be logged on to the chat room at the same time. This can be a particular problem for international courses where students may be working in different time zones and finding a mutually convenient time for the chat can be very difficult.

You will receive full instructions and guidance on how to log into the system you will be using and navigate around it just before your course starts. This will often be sent to you by email.

The chat room window will tell you who is in the chat room and what their role is (see Figure 6.4). A message in the chat window will tell you when someone arrives in the chat room and also when they leave. This will give you an idea of who you are 'talking' to and who is likely to respond to your messages. This helps you to 'speak' directly to individuals by using their name in your message.

Most chat rooms have an area where messages are composed. This message appears on the writer's screen only while it is in the 'compose area'. When the writer clicks the send button or hits the return key on the keyboard, the

CHAR ROOM			
Participants (8)	**Role**	**Queue**	
Liz Smith	Tutor	-	[Liz Smith joined the Session] July 7 2006 09.15 am BST
Graham Jones	Student		Liz Smith: Hi everyone! Just letting you know I'm here and ready for our chat about the assignment. How are you all today? July 7 2006 09.16 am BST
Abigail Perry	Student		[Juan Rodriguez joined the session] July 7 2006 09.17 am BST
Juan Rodriguez	Student		
Jonathan Adams	Student		Juan Rodriguez: Hi Liz! Thanks for being here, I'm really keen to discuss the assignment for the module as I'm ready to get started on it now. July 7 2006 09.21 am BST
Rosie Luke	Student		Geeter Hassani: I think we are all feeling a bit anxious about the assignment. Its quite different and I haven't done anything like this before. Do you think you could give us some tips, Liz? July 7 2006 09.24 am BST
Geeter Hassani	Student		
Maria Fabbri	Student		Liz Smith: Absolutely! I think everyone is feeling a bit anxious about the assignment at the moment, but I am hoping to allay your fears in this online chat/tutorial. What are you worried about the most everyone? July 7 2006 09.25 am BST
			....
		Compose:	I'm worried about	SEND

Figure 6.4 A diagrammatic representation of Rosie Luke's chat window for an online tutorial

Source: adapted from Simpson 2002: 103

message will then appear in the main window for everyone who is logged on to see. This gives you an opportunity to review what you have written and make any corrections and changes before you make your contribution.

One of the biggest difficulties with online chats is the speed at which you are able to type. If you are a slow typist it can take you a while to type a message and the conversation has already moved on before you make your contribution. Some chat rooms have a system whereby a student can click a button, which is the equivalent of putting their hand up so that the system puts them in a queue to speak.

Some online chats are archived – they can be saved and reviewed at a later date, which can be quite useful if you want to revisit the conversation later, but it means that what you say will be remembered so it's important to consider the rules of polite communication.

Box 6.2 gives an example of a chat room conversation between two students and a tutor that took place synchronously.

Here are some tips for working in chat rooms:

• Initially it's a good idea to keep the number of people you are trying to converse with at any one time to a maximum of around four. Too many people will make everything seem like it's happening too quickly, especially if you don't type very quickly.

Box 6.2

Chat room conversation

Liz said: Hi everyone. It's nice to see you all logged on. The aim of this online chat is to use it as a kind of tutorial to discuss the assignment. How are you getting on with it?

Helen said: I'm finding it a bit of a struggle to get started. Trying to analyse my own leadership qualities is quite difficult and I've never had to do it before.

Samir said: Yeah, Helen, I agree – all this is quite difficult. I haven't had to think about myself as a leader before and I find it hard to try to visualise how others see me!

Liz said: Yes a lot of people find that difficult. Once you get started it gets easier though. You might want to sit down and think about your strengths and weaknesses in terms of your interaction with others in the workplace, but I agree it's quite difficult to visualise how others see you. It's not really about that, it's about how you think you perform in terms of leading others and then you can compare that to feedback from others later.

Helen said: I see. So you want me to think about how I see myself rather than what I think others think?

Liz said: Exactly. Even that's not that easy, but it helps you to focus on something to begin with.

Samir said: This is really about reflection then?

- Make sure you set some ground rules with your colleagues about appropriateness of language and other stylistic matters. You could decide to make a statement about ignoring spelling mistakes and typographical errors – a common feature of most chat rooms. Think about how you will deal with stereotyping and discrimination in group members' postings, for example, and what language is deemed inappropriate for your group.
- Address people directly and by name if you are trying to make a point that is specifically relevant to them, or if you are asking them a question. Tutors will often do this when they want to get a specific student involved in the conversation.
- Don't stay in the chat room too long as it can be quite wearing. Tell people how long you are planning to stay and say goodbye when you leave.
- Say hello and goodbye when you arrive and leave the chat room – it helps others to notice you are there and encourages them to include you in the conversation.

- If there is somewhere in the VLE that you can post a picture of yourself try to do so (as well as provide some information that marks you out as an individual) – this, and similar postings from your colleagues, will help you to socialize online.

If you are using chat rooms outside of your place of work or educational institutions, access is less likely to be controlled. You need, then, to make sure that you practise safe chat room practice. Thames Valley Police, for example, provide some useful tips on this at: http://www.thamesvalley.police.uk/chatsafe/young.htm.

You can also access free chat rooms through a number of worldwide providers. These are often called 'messenger' services – some of the best known examples are 'MSN messenger' (http://messenger.msn.com) and 'Yahoo! Messenger' (http://messenger.yahoo.com). These providers offer software that you can download onto your computer for free and update regularly. You can invite friends and colleagues to join your group. These kinds of chat rooms tend to be used for less education-focused activities, but can be a fun way of staying in touch with people across the globe. Facilities such as these can also be very useful in supporting patients and clients online and providing health promotion activities with a variety of groups – especially young people who are most likely to be used to communicating in these ways (Rhodes 2004).

Making the most of working in a VLE

If you have any technical or other access problems, your tutor should be your first port of call and they will be able to seek additional technical advice if it is needed. It is important to remember that you may have access problems at first and that these are often easily resolved by the people who are there to support you. No matter how frustrating this may seem there is always a solution, but you may need help to get over this first hurdle. Don't try to struggle on – access your tutor by email or phone if you need help. Otherwise you won't get onto the first rung of the ladder in online learning.

Most virtual learning environments work in very much the same way as a website. The navigation, by clicking on buttons and links, is essentially the same, so if you can get used to surfing around an online supermarket or bookstore, then it's likely you won't find using a VLE very difficult.

VLEs are sharing tools, not data storage systems, so it is really important that you make sure that any work you place in shared folders in the VLE is backed up in some way. This is especially important if the work you have placed on the system is related to your assessment. There is always a real risk that a technical problem with the system can lead to the loss of files. These are easy to reload once the problem has been solved, providing you have kept a copy. If you haven't kept a copy then it might mean starting from scratch.

That's extremely frustrating if you have put a great deal of time and effort into creating the original document or text.

VLEs are designed to be easy to use and are meant to be student-friendly. However, just like any other piece of computer software, there will often be many features of the VLE of which you are not aware. Your tutor should provide you with a guide to your VLE that sets out some of the main features and should give you tips on how to use the VLE to your advantage.

As will be discussed in Chapter 9, when working online it is important to remember that most of your communication with others will be text based. Consequently, those who are communicating with you cannot see your face (unless, of course, you are using a web cam!) and the usual non-verbal cues are not present. Because of this, it is important to remember that the way in which you construct your emails and discussion board and chat room postings can easily lead to misunderstandings and hurt feelings if you are not careful.

Humour is quite an important aspect of everyday communication. It is often used by health and social care professionals with patients and clients with a view to injecting some informality into relationships and communication. The important thing to remember is that humour is often misunderstood, even in face-to-face situations where facial expressions can be used to supplement humorous language to ensure that the receiver understands the 'joke'. In online conversations, the problems of understanding or misunderstanding the joke can be quite damaging to group dynamics.

Emoticons are one way to include emotional expression in your postings. These are typed characters that often use keyboard characters to give the impression of facial expressions, to indicate an emotion or attitude, as to indicate intended humour. There are also some abbreviations used to express emotions, which are also commonly used in mobile telephone text messaging. Box 6.3 has some basic examples.

Box 6.3

Some common 'emoticons'/text abbreviations

:-)	Smile (indicating pleasure or joking)
:-(	Frown (indicating sadness or displeasure)
LOL	Laughs out loud!
;-)	Wink
:-D	Big smile
:-O	Mouth open in amazement

There are many more of these which you will find easily through a web search if you are interested.

Grammar, punctuation and spelling are sometimes an issue of contention when working in discussion boards and chat rooms and with email. On the whole, there is a degree of tolerance of some spelling and typographical errors – especially in chat rooms where students and tutor will type quite quickly and often make mistakes. **Text language** is a fast developing approach to writing mobile phone text messages to make the process of writing the message quicker. The use of this language should be discouraged in online discussion forums and chat rooms for education purposes as it is not always clear what is meant and not all users will understand the shorthand in use (see Activity 6.2).

Activity 6.2

Ground rules

Many tutors will ask new groups who are working together in the online environment to use a discussion forum to negotiate a set of group 'ground rules'.

Make some notes about the kinds of 'ground rules' you think are important to you in terms of how you expect others and yourself to behave. What is important to you?

Conclusion

Working in discussion boards and chat rooms can be immense fun and really enhance learning once you get used to it. Setting some specific time aside to undertake this activity is essential if you are to be a successful e-learner. Once you get used to it, working in discussion forums and chat rooms can become quite natural for you. There are, however, some pitfalls and ground rules that you need to bear in mind.

References

Clarke, A. (2004) *E-learning Skills*. Basingstoke: Palgrave.

Downing, K. and Chim, T.M. (2004) Reflectors as online extraverts? *Educational Studies* 30 (3): 265–276.

Kennedy, D.M. (2005) Standards for online teaching: lessons from the education, health and IT sectors. *Nurse Education Today* 25 (1): 23–30.

Lewis, D. and Allan B. (2005) *Virtual Learning Communities: A Guide for Practitioners*. Maidenhead: The Society for Research into Higher Education and Open University Press.

Rhodes, S.D. (2004) Hookups or health promotion? An exploratory study of chat room-based HIV prevention intervention for men who have sex with men. *AIDS Education and Prevention* 16 (4): 315–327.

Salmon, G. (2003) *E-moderating: The Key to Teaching and Learning Online*. London: Routledge Falmer.

Simpson, O. (2002) *Supporting Students in Online, Open and Distance Learning*, 2nd edition. London: Kogan Page.

Sit, J.H., Chung, J.W., Chow, M.C. and Wong, T.K. (2005) Experiences of online learning: students' perspective. *Nurse Education Today* 25 (2): 140–147.

Recommended further reading

Chellen, S. (2003) *The Essential Guide to the Internet for Health Professionals*. London: Routledge.

Clarke, A. (2004) *E-learning Skills*. Basingstoke: Palgrave.

7 Learning objects

Introduction

One aspect of e-learning is for students to work independently or as part of a group with online pages, multimedia and written material. This chapter briefly explains some of these options and outlines how they might work for you. There are many examples of this kind of activity, and we provide just a few of them here.

Learning materials

Learning materials are a central part of e-learning. Put simply, they are reusable bits of learning content. The learning objects, or materials, that you use during e-learning programmes can take a wide variety of forms and can serve several purposes (Clark 2004: 117). Examples of learning objects include multimedia content, instructional content, learning objectives, instructional software and software tools and any material that is designed to support student learning (Sloep 2004: 139, 141). The main aim of using these types of materials is to vary the approaches taken to learning so that students remain motivated and stimulated, and to bring learning alive by relating it to everyday practice in the student's workplace. These materials can be used both on their own and as part of an online activity with a online discussion or chat to follow. It is important to remember that successful learning online is likely to come from a combination of online communication and sharing with your fellow students, and the use of online learning materials and objects. One is unlikely to be successful without the other. Online learning that uses only interactive computer packages is usually called computer-based training and does not include the communication and sharing element.

Clark (2004: 114–116) offers the following list of possible types of learning materials. It is worth you knowing about these and what the issues are likely to be surrounding their use:

- study guides
- course websites
- World Wide Web

- interactive computer-based materials, such as interactive quizzes and CD-Roms
- open learning packs
- textbooks
- lecture notes
- reading lists
- presentations (including PowerPoint®)
- videos, video demonstrations and video lectures
- case studies and simulations
- problem-based learning scenarios
- case studies
- screen captures.

In this chapter we will try to illuminate for you how some of these materials might relate to your own learning. It is important to acknowledge that some students will be undertaking courses of study that are blended learning in the sense that face-to-face modes of delivery, such as lectures and seminars, are incorporated into the course along with electronic modes.

Course documents

If you are studying an e-learning course or module, it is likely that your course tutors will have created a variety of documents to enable you to familiarize yourself with the course content. These will include guides to the course and module that will contain a significant amount of material explaining how the course works and what the assessment will be. Sometimes they also contain a significant amount of learning material as well.

These documents will also most likely contain reading lists with references to articles, reports and books that will be useful in your learning. There may be a list of websites and it is well worth your visiting them, especially since they have been identified by your course tutors and so it is likely that they will be of some value and of good quality. For the most part, these documents will be sent to you by email, or be downloadable from the virtual learning environment or course web pages; occasionally you may receive them by post. In some instances your educational institution may send you a printed copy of the most essential documents by post. It is essential that you use these materials to inform your studies as much as you can. A great deal of time and effort will have gone in to making them a useful resource for you.

Games and quizzes

Most virtual learning environments provide tools that enable your tutors to create online games and quizzes. These can range from simple quizzes where you click buttons to answer multiple-choice answers and you are given feedback on your answers. Other options include short-answer, jumbled-sentence, crossword and matching/ordering questions. These games and quizzes often seem simplistic, but work on the principle that learning should be fun and they are a different and very useful way of checking your knowledge and understanding. They also help to vary the learning styles to meet different needs of different students and can be stimulating. Some systems will allow you to have multiple attempts at answering the questions so that you learn by previous mistakes. On the whole, online quizzes are simple to use. They offer you the opportunity to test your knowledge and are worth the effort of returning to regularly to check how you are progressing (see Activity 7.1).

Case studies and problem-based learning scenarios

Case studies have always been an important way of learning in health and social care. They help students to identify with real life situations and give them the opportunities to discuss the issues involved. They also assist in dealing with issues such as attitudes, stereotyping and discrimination by offering students the opportunity to consider some of the issues raised in society. They are likely to be a feature of online activities that will lead to discussions with your tutor and fellow students.

Problem-based learning (PBL) is an approach to learning that has spread around the world since the 1970s (Savin-Baden 2000). The principal idea behind PBL is that the trigger point for learning should be a problem, a query or a puzzle that the learner wishes to solve (Boud and Felettie 1991). Problem-based learning is now a popular way in health and social care education of using case-based or patient-focused scenarios, particularly in trying to maximize the effectiveness of interprofessional education across health and

Activity 7.1

Online games and quizzes

The Skills4Study website has a number of interactive quizzes and games for you to try.

Log on to the site at www.skills4study.com and click on either of the following:

- Games – this will take you to pages with a host of study skills related games to play.
- MP3 (audio files) – this will take you to a choice of audio clips about specific aspects of study skills for you to listen to.

social care staff (Reynolds 2003). This approach relies on the availability of realistic scenarios on which students can work in groups in order to develop skills in problem-solving and understand the issues around the scenario in question (Ward and Hartley 2006). As well as being realistic, problem-based learning scenarios also tend to be relatively vague so that students can identify their own learning needs in relation to the issues and this is what sets them apart from the usual case studies. Box 7.1 is an example of a fairly detailed case study based on an imaginary case used in child protection training. This might be used in problem-based learning.

Box 7.1

Example of a problem-based learning scenario from an online 'virtual family' related to an online workshop about child protection

The Briggs family
Dave Briggs – 34 years old
June Briggs – 33 years old
Billy Briggs – 8 years old
Chloe Briggs – 5 years old
Kylie Briggs – 3 years old
Roxanne Briggs – 18 months old

The family are of white English background. Both Dave and June come from large families, and both families have been known to Social Services because of concerns regarding the parents' capability to parent. June had spent some time in the care of the local authority, both in the children's units and foster homes. These arrangements were always on a voluntary basis when her parents were unable to cope with the demands of six children.

Social Services have had ongoing involvement with this family since the birth of Chloe. The children's names have been on the register on two occasions. The first time was when, following the birth of Chloe, there were concerns that she was failing to thrive for non-organic reasons and Billy was being neglected. The children were de-registered six months later when it was believed the situation had improved and the family would accept ongoing support. The second registration occurred two years ago when Billy was physically abused by Dave, who hit him with a leather belt for a minor misdemeanour. The other children were registered under the 'likely to be suffering from neglect' category.

Billy is presenting with behavioural difficulties at school and will often arrive at school hungry and dirty. He also appears to play a

---

significant role in looking after his siblings. Chloe is very isolated at school with no friends. She has been diagnosed as being short sighted, but does not come to school with her glasses. Kylie is currently at nursery. Her hygiene is also a problem and she appears to have speech and possible hearing difficulties. Roxanne has not been taken for any of her statutory health checks with the health visitor.

Dave is currently unemployed. It is believed that he drinks heavily on a daily basis and becomes violent when drunk, especially towards June. June is pregnant again. Without forethought or hesitation, Dave indulges his increasingly hedonistic impulses to spend, play and party, and is not deterred by anything or anyone. In addition to the daily uncertainty about Dave's state of mind, safety and mercurial attitude, there have been many desperate arguments between family members. Family members find it easier to believe that other people must be the cause of all of Dave's troubles than to dare consider that he has a 'shameful', 'frightening' mental illness.

Students would be asked to consider the scenario presented in Box 7.1 and their first step would be to work on some objectives for finding out more about the issues involved.

Another example of this approach is in the work of Sharp and Primrose (2003) and Ward and Hartley (2006), who have used online fictional families to create scenarios in a nursing programme. The 'Penfield Virtual Hospital' (www.hud.ac.uk/hhs/departments/nursing/penfield_site) is another example of a computer-based learning tool. It was developed by the University of Huddersfield, UK, for health care professionals and has used real case histories to provide the context to a learning tool that simulates the care context for patients within the environmental context of a general hospital.

Some universities and colleges are also now taking the trouble to create web pages that contain information about imaginary communities and towns to bring case histories and scenarios to life. For example the University of Wolverhampton is developing a multimedia 'online town' called New Molton at www.wlv.ac.uk/molt (see Figure 7.1). The site is used with health and social care students as well those studying law.

Simulated learning

Simulated learning is the process of imitating a real situation in order to provide students with an experience as close to the real one as possible so that they may learn about that situation and practise a series of skills.

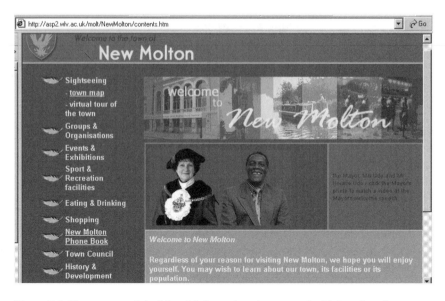

Figure 7.1 Home page of the New Molton virtual town at the University of Wolverhampton

Computers and the Internet can be used to simulate real life situations by using the same principles used to create computer games (computer animation) or graphics such as that used in film production. Classic examples are the flight simulators used to train airplane pilots. These technologies have already been harnessed in medicine to teach medical procedures such as laproscopic surgery and trauma life support. It is worth noting that, although these kinds of simulations are excellent learning tools, they are difficult to produce, requiring considerable technical skills, and can be expensive (Maier and Warren 2000: 54) so it is most likely your educational institution will have restricted the number it purchases or develops. Many of these simulations involve the use of a computer system to create lifelike symptoms and reactions in a manikin. These have been used for some time, for example, to teach resuscitation skills in health care. Often, the patient's data are used to create situations that are as lifelike as possible. Many of these approaches test the student's judgements, reactions and skills in a simulated, but close to reality, clinical situation. Such opportunities for learning and assessment, although using computer technology, are often classroom or clinical environment based. They allow students to practise skills in an environment where they can make decisions in similar situations to practice but without the danger of those decisions causing harm in real life.

Another approach to simulated learning is the use of role play. This is particularly useful in the development of the 'softer' skills of health and social care such as interviews, dealing with difficult communication situations such as giving bad news, and counselling. Education staff or even actors can be employed to play the part of patients and clients, giving the student the opportunity to work in a situation which feels as real as possible. Often, situations can be videoed to enable the student to receive feedback and discuss with their tutor their performance, progress and need for further learning. Facilities such as learning laboratories, clinical skills facilities and communication suites on campuses and in practice settings are commonly used for this purpose.

Sometimes it is possible to translate these ideas into an online environment, particularly where communications skills are concerned, by using the discussion board or chat room. See the example in Box 7.2.

Video material

Computers can be used to record and store audio and video as digital files. Video material has been used for many years in teaching health and social care

---

Box 7.2

Simulated learning

Here is an example of how simulated learning can operate in an online environment.

Sam was undertaking an online course in social care for people with mental health problems. The focus of the module he was currently undertaking was on depression and anxiety. At the end of the module the tutor had planned an online discussion with the students using the discussion boards.

The tutor acted the part of a depressed individual, John, who was seeking support from an online discussion forum during one evening.

Students were aware of the existing guidance for assessing and managing depression and had been given material to study prior to the online session. The idea was for the students to support the individual through an online discussion forum that took place in real time.

The tutor placed pressure on the students by posting messages indicating John's distress, posting things such as: '. . . you don't seem to be responding to the things I am saying very quickly, are you still there?' and '. . . I really feel like ending it all right now'.

The session lasted for 30 minutes, which is quite a long time to be working in an online discussion or chat room constantly. The students' evaluation, however, was mostly positive in that they found the experience of working in a pressurized environment with 'live' issues very stimulating.

students. These are often used in classroom teaching to illustrate issues and bring them to life. The advent of the Internet and digital media now allows the delivery of video material electronically either on a CD or DVD (digital video data) or via the Internet. Delivery of video material via the Internet is known as **video streaming**. This means that students can view videos by clicking on a **hyperlink** and the download is progressive. They do not actually need to completely download the video before it begins playing; it starts almost as soon as the click has been made (Green et al. 2003). With the development of better quality Internet connections and video media, the wealth of material that can be delivered online is immense.

The most obvious use of video in e-learning is in the video lecture where 'key' subject areas are delivered in the classroom and are videoed for live delivery on the Internet or, more likely, as a **pod cast** for future use. This helps to provide a link with the traditional learning methods which suit some students' learning styles. A tutor can be available online via a discussion forum or chat room to discuss the issues once the video has been viewed. Students will often be asked to watch a video and then complete an online assessment of what they have learnt from it. Some of the possibilities are:

- practical demonstrations
- real life and simulated practical situations of clients and patients
- case studies
- testimonials
- lectures and speeches
- documentary films.

In order to benefit from this form of learning material you will need to ensure that you have the correct software to play videos.

If you are using DVD or CD-Rom video material you will need a CD reader in your computer and software that allows the playing of DVDs. There are a large number of pieces of software that do this:

- Quick Time Player (www.apple.com/quicktime/win.html)
- Real Player (http://uk.real.com/)
- Windows Media Player (www.microsoft.com/windows/windowsmedia).

Another useful site is at www.download.com where a variety of free software as well as music and video are available for download. Click on the link to software and then audio and video. Some of these systems often come ready loaded on your computer, but basic versions can also be downloaded free from the Internet from the links above. The same facilities are also used for playing music online and listening to online radio stations.

In order to listen to video and audio material it is also important to remember that you need either integral or separate speakers and the software

Activity 7.2

Stanford Health Library online video collection

The Stanford Health Library at http://healthlibrary.stanford.edu/
resources/videos.html (accessed 24 August 2006) offers a number of
videos about a variety of aspects of health, many of which are lectures.
(The site also offers a link to the download of 'real player'.)

Visit the site and click on one of the links to a subject of interest to you.
There are a number of topic areas of interest to social care professionals
as well as health care. Some of the quality is not perfect, but the videos
on offer will give you an idea of how this works. You might need to
remember to enable your pop-ups to make the best of this media.

Make some notes about what you think of the video material
available here. Are there ways that you think it can be improved? In
what ways was it useful to you?

needed to provide sound. Once again, most new computers come with these
facilities. Activity 7.2 gives an example of an online video library.

CD-Rom interactive and multimedia packages

Multimedia is a concept within the computer world that means the use of
various types of media including sound, images, animation, video and text.
The term 'interactive' signifies that you have some kind of interaction with
the material in the package rather than just passively watching, listening to,
looking at or reading it. This encourages learner participation and activates
learning. The advantage of this kind of material is that you are usually able
to work through the package at your own pace.

Multimedia packages can be delivered online via the Internet or a virtual
learning environment, but most commonly are packaged on to a compact
disc known as a CD-Rom. These facilities tend to start up themselves when
they are placed into the CD drawer (or D: Drive) of your computer. The media
can be 'read' by you but not altered. The advantage of using a CD for this is
that it does not require an Internet connection. CDs containing multimedia
tend to need quite a large amount of computer space and download speed can
be quite slow from the Internet. They are relatively inexpensive to send
through the post.

The media, for example, might include some text, introducing the students
to the contents of the package or programme. There will also be a menu,
outlining what is contained within the package and allowing the student to

---

Box 7.3

Online multimedia at the BBC

There are numerous online multimedia packages available on the Internet. There are many good examples available on the BBC website. For example, try the following link: http://www.bbc.co.uk/health/interactive_area/. Here you will find examples of a variety of media such as courses, quizzes and games related to health topics of value to the general population.

---

move backwards and forwards between one section of the package and another. Box 7.3 illustrates one example of online multimedia.

Conclusion

There are a wide variety of ways in which learning materials can be created and delivered online. A mixed, hybrid approach to learning which includes interactive materials as well as other text-based options and online interaction help to motivate students and to meet a wide variety of learning styles. Your course may well offer you the opportunity to interact with a variety of interactive ideas and materials. We have offered a number of examples in this chapter for you to think about. More and more realistic materials will undoubtedly be available in the future, constrained only by imagination and by the ability of your computer.

References

Boud, D. and Feletti, G. (eds) (1991) *The Challenge of Problem Based Learning*. London: Kogan Page.

Clark, A. (2004) *E-learning Skills*. Basingstoke: Palgrave.

Green, S., Voegeli, D., Harrison, M., Phillips, J., Knowles, J., Weaver, M. and Shepard, K. (2003) Evaluating the use of streaming video to support student learning in a first-year life sciences course for student nurses. *Nurse Education Today* 23 (4): 255–261.

Maier, P. and Warren, A. (2000) *Integrating Technology in Learning and Teaching: A Practical Guide for Educators*. London: Kogan Page.

Reynolds, F. (2003) Initial experiences of interprofessional problem-based learning: a comparison of male and female students' views. *Journal of Interprofessional Care* 17 (1): 35–42.

Savin-Baden, S. (2000) *Problem Based Learning in Higher Education: Untold Stories*. Buckingham: Open University Press.

Sharp, D.M. and Primrose, C.S. (2003) The 'virtual family': an evaluation of an innovative approach using problem-based learning to integrate curriculum themes in a nursing undergraduate programme. *Nurse Education Today* 23 (3): 219–225.

Sloep, P. (2004) Learning objects: are they the answer to the knowledge economy's predicament? In: Jochems, W., Van Merrienboer, J. and Koper, R. (eds) *Integrated E-learning: Implications for Pedagogy, Technology and Organisation*. London: Routledge.

Ward, K. and Hartley, J. (2006) Using a virtual learning environment to address one problem with problem based learning. *Nurse Education in Practice* 6 (4): 85–191.

8 Working in online communities

Introduction

The principle of online learning communities and communities of practice lends itself well to health and social care practice. The aim of this chapter is to explore the potential of this in health and social care online education.

What are online communities?

The majority of us are familiar with the notion of formal, classroom or clinical learning. In health and social care, however, over the years there has been a distinct shift from a didactic approach to teaching to a more adult model of learning. In addition to the shift to adult learning, with its emphasis on the experience being more student led, there has also been a growing interest in professional development that meets the needs of practice and encourages a problem-solving approach. This is not unique to health and social care; Lewis and Allan (2005: 5) allude to the 'paradigm shift' as existing in higher education generally. They describe 'learning communities' as being 'groups of professionals and practitioners, often from the same or related professional background' (Lewis and Allan 2005: 6). The learning communities come together to share knowledge and experience and solve work-related problems. In solving the work-related problems, participants also gain in knowledge and therefore develop as practitioners. Wilson and Ryder (1996) suggest that learning communities involve shared control and transformative communication where everyone participates in the learning experience. The idea of a learning community, therefore, is a group of people with a common professional interest who share knowledge and experience, and learn together as a means to solve particular work-based problems (see Box 8.1).

Communities of practice

Wenger and colleagues (2002: 4) describe 'communities of practice' in a similar way to online communities, where participants 'share a concern, a set of problems, or a passion about a topic, and who deepen their knowledge and

---

Box 8.1

Learning communities

Members have

- shared or similar professional background
- shared set of interests and problems
- commitment to the generation of shared and new knowledge.

---

expertise in this area by interacting on an ongoing basis.' They also suggest that communities of practice are not a new idea. They argue that they exist in all aspects of life – both professional and social. This notion rests on a social theory of learning based on observation of work-based learning in different professional groups by Lave and Wenger (1991). They suggest that many of these communities are informal and are unrecognized by employers. Social communities in this context would arise out of a mutual passion for a particular area of interest such as a hobby or a particular genre of music whereas professional communities would be entirely work related (see Activity 8.1).

The terminology relating to communities of learning varies. Lewis and Allan (2005) describe 'learning community' as a generic term that encompasses all collaborative learning groups. Lave and Wenger (1991) discuss 'communities of practice' in relation to work-based learning. Lewis and Allan (2005) also allude to 'communities of interest', which they describe as being large groups or networks that share and disseminate information rather than being related to learning per se. This chapter will use the term 'communities of practice', because this identifies the work-related learning that is central to health and social care, practice being a term that is familiar to those who work within this field in whatever context they work.

Activity 8.1

Identifying a community of practice

Try to identify at least one community of practice you may be involved in, whether this is in your social or professional life.

What set of interests and/or problems do the members of the community share?

Is it a formal or informal group?

Online communities of practice are as described above, only the medium of their knowledge exchange and problem-solving is a Virtual Learning Environment rather than a classroom or meeting room. The online nature of these communities of practice allows practitioners from a local, national or even international background to participate. Online communities of practice can utilize a range of communication tools such as email, discussion boards, chat rooms and virtual classrooms and this facilitates a flexible approach to collaborative learning. Methods of communication within online communities will be discussed later in this chapter.

Who can participate in an online community of practice?

A community of practice can arise as part of a formal learning experience such as a module within a programme of study specifically set up to encourage collaborative learning on a specific topic. They can also arise out of a specific clinical issue or problem, which is not related to formal learning. The formal learning approach will determine some of the characteristics of the participants but the pure work-based approach can be more open in respect of membership. As identified above the members of the group need to have a shared or similar professional background. This does not mean they all have to be 'qualified' practitioners nor does it mean they all have to have the same overall professional interest, for example physiotherapy, radiography or nursing. What it does mean is the need to have a shared interest in a specific area of care, for example child protection, care of the adult with learning disabilities in the community, prevention of falls or Alzheimer's disease. The topic area therefore determines the make-up of the community in terms of the staff groups involved. The make-up of the community should match the multidisciplinary team associated with the subject matter, for example child protection involves a number of professionals such as social workers, paediatricians, health visitors and accident and emergency practitioners. The community can be a local one or it can encompass either national or international membership. This element of the community will, again to some extent, be determined by the nature of the issue, which gave rise to it in the first place. The issue may be a purely local one or may be something, which has distinct national or international overtones. International links in health and social care are becoming more relevant as issues become global; this is particularly true in respect of infectious diseases which spread across the world rapidly as a result of increased transcontinental travel, as evidenced in the SARS epidemic.

The vital element of a community of practice is that members must have a common focus and an incentive to work together (Wilson and Ryder 1996). This common focus can transcend the usual geographical barriers and learning can be considerably enhanced by sharing a more global view of the issue or problem. For example, a community of practice relating to traumatic wound management could include practitioners from the armed forces medical services and countries where there is or has been war or natural disaster as well as practitioners from an acute hospital service in a specific locality. A similar example would be an international approach to a community of practice relating to HIV and AIDS where practitioners in Africa for instance have a wealth of knowledge to share with developed-world workers who can share new treatments and research findings with their African counterparts. A community of practice needn't benefit only from 'experts' on a topic; it is also worth bearing in mind that they can benefit from novice members who bring a fresh view on the issues while learning (see Activity 8.2). Some issues that practitioners may wish to learn collaboratively about may be so uncommon as to necessitate a more global group to ensure that the community is wide enough to share knowledge, for example a group of practitioners interested in a rare disease or syndrome or a new technique.

Lewis and Allan (2005) suggest that communities should be relatively small and Wenger et al. (2002), in emphasizing the social nature of the learning, appear to concur with this. Since the interaction online requires a level of trust and confidence in one another and yet sufficient numbers to ensure lively discussion and debate then Lewis and Allan's (2005) suggestion of between 6 and 24 people would seem realistic. Fewer than 6 and there is limited scope for debate and shared learning; more than 24 and online interaction becomes unwieldy and relationships can become too superficial and subgroups can appear. The subject area can define the actual number or if it is part of a formalized learning process it may be determined by the numbers applying to join. Some communities of practice may be larger overall but these tend to divide into smaller groups to manage the learning experience.

Interprofessional education is high on the health and social care agenda currently as the boundaries between professional groups are blurring and new roles are being developed to meet specific resource deficits. There is a growing recognition that the traditional approaches are not sustainable and that a high quality service requires a range of different practitioners who can provide flexible and user friendly care. This has brought with it recognition that no one practitioner can function in isolation but that patient or client needs often require a range of skills and knowledge. Communities of practice

Activity 8.2

Issues and problems in a community of practice

Think of issues and/or problems from your sphere of practice that could be the focus of a community of practice.

Are the issues and/or problems you have identified local or could they benefit from a national or even international community of practice approach?

can address the interprofessional education element by including all those practitioners with an interest in the subject matter as highlighted above. This could include both qualified and unqualified and may even include service users depending on the nature of the issue or problem (see Activity 8.3).

Lewis and Allan (2005) propose some examples of the types of groups who could form a learning community. These can be adapted to health and social care as follows:

- professional teams – these could be uni- or multi-professional in nature
- multi-professional teams working on improving services or developing practice
- interdisciplinary teams working on developing cutting-edge techniques or research
- special interest groups
- practitioners working across traditional boundaries.

It could be argued that the most common approach would be the team working to improve services or develop practice; however, there is some applicability in the other approaches.

What is essential to the formation of a community of practice is the commitment to the community and a passion for the subject area. It requires time and energy to form and develop a community of practice and even then it may not work (Wenger et al. 2002).

Benefits of communities of practice

There are many benefits from the formation and development of communities of practice. These benefits can be both tangible and less obvious in nature, short and long term. There are benefits for the individuals involved, the organizations associated with those individuals and for practice generally. This section will therefore discuss these benefits from the perspective of health and social care.

Activity 8.3

Groups in a community of practice

Using the examples you thought of in the previous activity, consider the different groups of staff who may be part of the community of practice for each issue/problem you listed.

Think about what you would be able to learn from each group of staff in broad terms even before you began to address more focused learning in respect of the issue/problem.

Wenger et al. (2002) discuss tangible and intangible value in respect of communities of practice. They allude to the tangible products of learning i.e. increased knowledge and/or skills and the improved standards associated with these. They also acknowledge that there are less tangible benefits such as the new or improved relationships, the increased confidence and ability to be innovative and the sense of belonging that arise from the process. Arguably these benefits would also arise from more traditional means of learning; however, it can also be seen that the shared control and the need to collaborate would enhance the less tangible benefits. It is possible to sit in a classroom session and have no interaction with other members of the student group at all and only limited interaction with the teacher. In an online community of practice this can still occur, but generally it is less likely because of the nature of the approach. To a certain extent, it is possible that the relative anonymity of the online environment actually enhances participation and therefore a sense of belonging. This would seem somewhat incongruous but it is sometimes the difficulty of being heard or the problems of shyness that negatively affect interaction in a classroom. Online, however, these things are not always such a problem. Indeed, it is possible that participation in an online community of practice could markedly improve a practitioner's overall confidence and thereby improve their overall performance in practice.

The practitioner benefits are perhaps the more obvious outcomes of the community of practice approach to learning. There are both short-term and long-term benefits for the individual and include the following:

- access to expertise
- sharing of knowledge and skills
- help with problems and challenges
- sense of professional identity
- network for information exchange.

The access to expertise is an obvious benefit to the practitioner who is starting out; however, it is also true that in health and social care, learning is lifelong. It does not matter how experienced you may be, there is always some aspect of clinical knowledge you do not have. The sharing of knowledge and skills is always of value in practice to ensure that care is evidence based and of the highest possible quality. There has been a shift towards the sharing of 'best practice' to improve overall quality of service delivery and communities of practice can provide a forum for this, although this is not the primary aim. The exchange of information is somewhat different from sharing of knowledge and may not be a learning experience as such. The information shared may not be of direct value or use, but is nevertheless worthwhile just to keep the practitioner abreast of current practice elsewhere. The networking is both a short-term and long-term benefit as relationships established in this manner can be sustained beyond the life of the community. A major benefit for the individual member however is the opportunity to interact with like-minded practitioners and discuss matters that they have a real passion for. There is a great deal of enjoyment to be had from being able to share your passion with others who have equal commitment and interest. There is also a sense of satisfaction and achievement to be had from helping to solve a practice-related problem, whether it is yours or someone else's. Each member can also gain a sense of belonging to a community that shares a common purpose and in which all have equal standing. This is a benefit that should not be underestimated because the pressures of work and the difficulties of creating an appropriate work–life balance can leave health and social care practitioners feeling isolated and lonely. Belonging to an online community of practice can reduce considerably this sense of isolation, despite the virtual nature of the contact.

The advantages to the organization revolve around having practitioners who are better informed, have enhanced knowledge and skills and an improved ability to problem solve. The community as a whole may be working towards solving a problem or issue that has significant relevance to the organization, and this has obvious benefits. The networking element of the community will have value to the organization as well as to the individual in that it presents opportunities to 'benchmark' practice against that in other similar organizations. A community of practice approach to learning means that practitioners are gaining skills and knowledge that are directly relevant to their roles. They are not tied to attending formal teaching at a given date and time but can be learning within the workplace and responding to 'real world' issues. The downside for the practitioner in relation to this may be limited time and access to computers. However, if the organization can perceive tangible benefits, the managers are more likely to be supportive of the process. One of the problems with professional development for staff is that it is often not always clear that there are direct benefits in terms of patient or client care. Communities of practice can demonstrate tangible value in respect of practice and practice development, thereby providing the evidence required to gain managerial support. This tangible evidence arises out of the close link between practice and the learning process that is the ethos of communities of practice.

The advantages to practice have already been highlighted under practitioner and organizational benefits. However, they should be emphasized because the potential for improved care is tremendous. The community can work together to bring a range of expertise and experience to bear on a problem or issue. Furthermore, the possibility of bringing a multidisciplinary approach to practice is of value, not only in terms of the problem itself, but also in bringing about greater understanding of different professional roles and contributions to care.

Models of online communities of practice

Lewis and Allan (2005) suggest that there are three models of virtual learning communities. The models reflect the needs of the members and their associated organizations, and the nature of their learning requirements. The models are:

- simple
- managed
- complex.

Lewis and Allan (2005) describe the simple community as being one which forms spontaneously because of the mutual interests and problems of the membership. These simple communities of practice can be small or large, and may have an open or closed membership (see Box 8.2).

The facilitator of the community may be someone who is self-appointed, selected by the membership or a role that is rotated. This type of community of practice may exist outside the formal structures of health and social care organizations. Members may be from the same organization, even the same department, or they may come together from different organizations and may cross professional and geographical boundaries.

Simple communities of practice are useful for providing a network for practitioners with a mutual professional interest. However, there is a danger that they can become a clique and that the focus is on the individuals' interests rather than the work-related issues. These negative aspects are not unique to online communities of practice but can occur in any grouping of people. Good facilitation can assist with avoiding or minimizing the problems and enhancing the advantages (see Box 8.3).

Managed communities of practice are supported by an organization or agency, such as a particular NHS Trust, Social Services area, a university or a professional organization. They may well be developed to address a particular strategic need or problem (see Box 8.4). Members of the community

---

Box 8.2

Simple communities of practice

- A small closed group of active members where the individuals in the group remain constant over time.
- A small open group where membership changes over time but there is a core of active members.
- A large closed group of members where the individuals involved change very little over time.
- A large open group where membership is fluid but there is a core of active members to maintain the group.

Box 8.3

Case study of an online community of practice for physiotherapists

Maria attended a traditional classroom-based course related to her role as a specialist respiratory care physiotherapist. She felt stimulated not only by the course content but also by the networking with colleagues from across the region who had similar roles to hers. In her NHS Trust she was the only physiotherapist who had a specialist respiratory medicine role and, although her colleagues from the Physiotherapy department and the ward staff she worked with were supportive and friendly, she often felt isolated in her role. During the course she attended an optional session on e-learning and the speaker mentioned online communities of practice. Maria reflected on this and asked the speaker to explain further after the session. At the end of the course, when the participants got together for a final coffee, Maria suggested that they could form an online community of practice to continue their networking, despite the geographical distribution of the group. Most were in favour of such a move. Maria got further advice from her NHS Trust information technology support department and set up a small community.

The online community of practice worked well and Maria and her colleagues were able to discuss work-related issues, help one another with problem-solving and generally support one another. Maria initially facilitated the community but then they agreed to rotate the role throughout the group.

Maria no longer felt isolated at work but instead was more motivated and confident in her role and developed the service she offered due to her renewed enthusiasm and ability to discuss her ideas with colleagues with a wide range of respiratory care experience.

---

may come from different organizations, not just the one that has initiated it. The process of establishing the community and guiding its activities is initially managed by the founding organization but this guidance will become less obvious as the community stabilizes and the problem-solving gets underway.

Complex communities are associated with organizational improvement or regional projects and may well involve a number of partnerships and affiliations to achieve their goals. The wide remit of these communities means that they are divided into smaller communities. These smaller communities then feed into a central community, which has responsibility for maintaining the overall focus and pulling all the pieces together into a whole. This approach to communities of practice is similar to the notion of having several

---

Box 8.4

Case study of a community of practice for teenage clients

Newtown Primary Care Trust (PCT) serves a community where there has been a high level of teenage pregnancy for some time. The PCT recognized the need to address this problem and decided to set up a community of practice online since there are a wide range of professional groups they needed to involve and not all of them belonged to Newtown PCT. A community of practice allowed them to access people with expertise from their own Trust, as well as the acute hospital Trust and Social Services, and enabled discussion and implementation of strategies to reduce teenage pregnancy and addressing of associated issues such as sexual health and general health education. A senior manager with some experience of information technology as well as health care took on the role of facilitator, while a group of managers from the PCT provided support and direction until the community was functioning independently.

Two years after it was set up, the community of practice had made real progress. Although the actual reduction in teenage pregnancy was small, there were much better links between primary and acute care and social services. Services were being developed to meet a wide range of health and health education needs of teenagers, particularly in relation to sexual health and family planning advice. There had also been considerable interest shown by the local education authority and the Council's Youth Services department, who felt that they could benefit from a similar approach, either separately or by joining the existing community.

The individual practitioners involved in the community felt that they had gained a lot from it. They had gained professional development but had also been able to gain assistance in solving problems. They were able to be more effective in providing care for their teenage clients.

---

working groups feeding information into a central committee as a means to getting a complex project completed. Each of the smaller groups functions as a simple community of practice except that they address issues related to the overall project and therefore provide feedback to the centre. There is still the same opportunity for learning for individuals as with other approaches to online communities of practice. The focus remains on practice but the overall aim is to address a strategic issue from a 'bigger picture' perspective rather than the more operational outlook of the simple communities and the single issue strategy of the managed model (see Box 8.5).

Box 8.5

Case study of a community of practice for critical care provision

The regional Critical Care Network identified that there was a need to coordinate education across its 'patch' because universities were discontinuing their courses due to low student numbers. There were clearly a number of issues that needed addressing including resourcing staff development, what education and training needs there were and how these could be delivered in a financially viable way. They also recognized that an associated problem was the need to improve standards of care in some units, and to create better links between all the services involved in critical care delivery to make care more effective. The biggest issue within this element of the problem was the care of children who required critical care. They often had to be placed on adult units where staff felt inadequately prepared to care for them. The network realized that solving these problems would involve a number of different partnerships and a range of professional groups needed to be brought together. An online community of practice approach was agreed on.

From the outset there was recognition that the 'project' was too big and complex for a single community of practice to deal with, so a complex community approach was selected with each smaller group being given the remit for a single aspect. Multi-professional communities were set up with membership from different organizations including higher education providers. The central group facilitated the whole project and was also made up of different professional and organizational groupings.

David, a staff nurse from an intensive care unit, was part of a community tasked with considering the education needs of staff from intensive care. He initially felt quite shy and did not contribute to the community, preferring to lurk in the discussions. However, he soon realized he had something to offer and that the other members were not at all intimidating. He began to enjoy belonging to the community and got a great deal of satisfaction when they arrived at a consensus view of a way forward. David learned a lot about the possibilities on offer from education providers and also why they sometimes seemed slow to respond to service needs. He also learned about how other professional colleagues perceived critical care provision and what the different professionals could learn from one another. At the same time he realized that he had contributed to the community in a way which enhanced others understanding of the nursing perspective and had personally provided a significant amount of information which others in the community had not previously known.

Communities of practice can also be used as a formal learning experience. An education provider facilitates these online communities and members work towards academic credits as well as considering a work-related issue. Because of the academic process involved, these communities are time limited. An academic year is usually a practical time frame, although there is nothing to prevent members maintaining the community beyond the educational element. This is a relatively new approach to communities of practice but is very much in keeping with the ethos of adult education, which enhances a practitioner's ability to undertake their role effectively. This type of online community is generally a simple one however it is possible for academic credit to be attached to the work of a small community that is part of a complex approach to communities of practice. This would need to be carefully thought out to ensure that the overall aim of the community did not compromise the educational element.

The life cycle of a community of practice

Lewis and Allan (2005) and Wenger et al. (2002) refer to a community of practice as a living, growing entity that goes through developmental stages. It is useful to understand these stages, both as a facilitator and a member, in order to allow the community to grow and the members to support each other through any associated problems. Although the two texts referred to above use slightly different terminology for the stages, fundamentally they are the same. Each community of practice will therefore go through the following stages:

- foundation
- induction
- incubation
- improving performance
- implementation
- closure or change.

These stages are not entirely dissimilar to the notion of team development. This is not surprising given that, as with any group, a community needs time to get to know one another and clarify roles and responsibilities before becoming effective in respect of their group aims. A community will have a time limit and will either discontinue or will change into a different entity to address different issues, possibly with new members.

Whether formed spontaneously, or set up as managed or complex communities to address a specific activity, communities of practice all need some time to develop the structure of the community – this is the foundation phase. This is the time when the following issues need to be considered:

- Purpose – what are the aims and objectives of the community?
- Structure – what model will be used for the community?

- Membership – who could potentially contribute to the aims and objectives of the community?
- How will the community function together to facilitate learning and working?
- What information and communication technology (ICT) is needed and how will the virtual learning environment work?
- Is any further support needed, e.g. administrative support?

The purpose of the community is an important aspect to consider, as it will determine many of the other points made above, particularly the potential membership. The purpose may be initially quite vague and broad, with a more focused approach evolving with the community; however, it is necessary to have an overall aim from the outset. The size of the community may be a factor to consider. Generally for learning and professional development to occur, the group needs to be quite small and it may be that where a larger number of members is identified more than one community is established. Wenger et al. (2002) do suggest that larger groups are possible; however, Lewis and Allan (2005) assert that smaller groups with fewer than 24 members are more effective. In health and social care, it is probably better to have more than one community rather than have a single large group where interaction is more formal. Some members may be inclined to simply lurk in a large community whereas in a smaller one they will feel more able to contribute to discussions.

The technical support for a community of practice is a very important consideration. The NHS and local authorities are constantly developing their ICT infrastructure but this remains problematical in some areas. There are sometimes problems with access to the Internet and even the computers for community members and systems between organizations may not be compatible. Therefore getting advice from the appropriate technical people is vital to ensure the success of a community.

The virtual learning environment needs to meet the community's needs and be user friendly because not all members will be confident with this medium of learning. It needs to be attractive and to take into account that some members may have a disability, such as dyslexia. Most of all, it should make you, the learner and community member, want to get involved. As part of getting members keen to be involved, there should be a process of welcome and introduction. You may be asked to provide a digital photograph and a mini-biography to place in a gallery of members.

The induction stage needs to be facilitated and this is when the community introduces itself and the individual members get to know one another (see Box 8.6). It is also a time for inducting members into the community so that they can participate. An online community may benefit from a face-to-face induction to get to know one another and to ensure everyone is familiar with the technology. Where this is not possible, the facilitator will need to find some other means of doing this, such as telephone conversations or online exercises to familiarize members with the virtual learning environment and each other. As an individual member, it is important that you participate in the induction phase because it will help you get the most out of the community and also help you contribute to it effectively. You may not always find the induction tasks appealing, particularly if icebreakers are used, and you may feel impatient to get on with the main business of the community. However, this period of time is important as it will help to develop relationships and thereby enhance the interactions, which are essential to achieving the aims. Socializing is central to any e-learning and is particularly so in communities of practice.

The setting of ground rules is also an important part of the induction of an online community of practice. As with any community, it is essential that everyone understands what is considered acceptable and what is not. In health and social care there are issues, such as confidentiality, that are a necessary rule. Frequency of online participation is an issue that the community has to agree to ensure that activities are not missed because expectations of members are unrealistic.

The incubation phase is when the community begins to interact and work together. This is the time when trust needs to develop and members begin to engage in discussion and debate. The facilitator will need to 'incubate' the community and actively encourage interaction. Trust is an essential element

---

Box 8.6

Example of a member's introduction

Hi Everyone,

I'm Helen and I am a social worker working with the palliative care team. I enjoy my job and have joined this community in the hope that I can gain knowledge and help with developing services in relation to palliative care for long term conditions as well as for those with cancer.

I am married to Robert and we have a nine month old baby boy, James, and two cats. I don't have a lot of spare time at the moment with the demands of a full time job and a baby but enjoy playing badminton and swimming.

I am looking forward to working and learning with you all.

Helen

of a community of practice; without discussion and debate, it will not properly develop and the aims of the community will not be met. The relationships in the community not only need to be trusting but also need to develop in order to allow for humour and fun so that your learning and problem-solving is enjoyable. There should be a sense of collective responsibility and co-dependency, because this will assist the community with sharing knowledge and expertise and helping with each other's problems (Lewis and Allan 2005). You need to be responsible for contributing your knowledge and expertise but you also need to be able to feel that you can ask for help from other members (see Box 8.7).

Phase four is improving performance. This is when the community starts to address its aims and objectives. At this time, members will be engrossed in their collaboration and interaction levels will be high. A sense of satisfaction and excitement can often be perceived as members see that progress is being made and they are learning new things and working together to address practice issues. This phase is followed by implementation when the work of the community has an impact on practice and changes occur both in practice and in the community members.

Box 8.7

Case study of a community of practice for obese clients

The Obesity Community of Practice is a group of interested practitioners who want to improve the advice and care provided for obese clients. The community includes practice nurses, health visitors, nutritionists and physiotherapists. They have been developing their relationships and sharing ideas and have recently decided to consider how to encourage healthy eating in clients with poor diet and low income. Collaboratively they have devised a scoring system for food that allows clients to earn treats for good eating behaviours. Although the physiotherapist has limited knowledge of the nutritional aspects of the scheme, he is a talented amateur artist and using the information provided to him has designed an attractive information sheet and poster to support the scheme. They piloted their programme of advice with some success.

The successful implementation of the community's new scheme gave them a real sense of satisfaction and encouraged them to continue to explore other means of helping obese clients. All felt that they had learned a lot from their community of practice participation and that, not only had a new scheme come from it, but also they had developed as practitioners.

Eventually a community may come to the end of its life, either as a result of achieving its goals or because it has evolved into a new community with new goals. Closure should be a part of the cycle and participants should reflect on the community's achievements and have the opportunity to formally end the community and say their goodbyes. Networks may continue beyond the life of the community either for work or social purposes. As at the induction of a community, a face-to-face final get-together may be helpful to celebrate the community and its achievements.

Communication in online communities of practice

Communication, and the socialization it creates, is central to the effective functioning of a community of practice. Virtual learning environments provide a range of means for communicating between members of a community (see Box 8.8). It is essential that each member understands the means of communication it is going to use and that there is guidance provided as to how each will be used to facilitate the business of the community.

Box 8.8

Communication tools

- Email – most people are familiar with email as a communication tool. Most learning environments will facilitate individual or group email postings. This is useful for sending information to the group, particularly when you want them to get it quickly because many people access their emails regularly.
- Virtual notice boards – as the name suggests, this is a means of posting notices or announcements. This tends to be used for news and informing the community of new resources etc. It is a means of updating the community with news.
- Discussion boards – again the name suggests the function of this communication method. This area is utilized for discussion and debate on relevant matters. New topics or threads can be introduced and the discussion is permanently visible to everyone in the community.
- Chat rooms – this allows synchronous communication and is useful for issues that need 'real time' discussion. They can be used for the more social aspects of the group and may enhance the sense of belonging. Where face-to-face induction cannot take place, this can be a useful means of getting to know one another.

Online communities of practice depend on communication and this is why the ground rules should include how often participation will take place. If discussion isn't frequent enough, it can become stagnant due to lack of debate, notices go unnoticed and motivation falls off. The ethos of a community is that members share knowledge and expertise; this can happen only if they communicate regularly and all members are committed to entering into discussion. This is particularly true with quite small communities where there is no allowance for lurking.

Using the methods of communication for social exchanges is also beneficial for the community. Exchanging recipes, commenting on books or films or simply telling others about anything that you feel is relevant will enhance the sense of belonging. You can start a discussion board for 'coffee shop' or similar conversation to provide a forum for this.

Conclusion

Online communities of practice are a means of enabling practitioners to learn and work together towards improving practice in an area of care they are all interested and involved in. This approach to online learning is congruent with a more work-based learning ethos that enables practitioners' personal, professional development to link closely with practice development. Communities of practice are also useful for facilitating interprofessional learning and helping different professional groups to understand each other better. Practitioners from a local, national or international arena can create an online community and the focus of their learning can be a particular area of interest, for example ophthalmics, care of the dying, dementia care or a practice or organizational problem, such as providing out-of-hours care, meeting the care needs of homeless people or falls prevention. Online communities of practice promote a collaborative approach to health and social care that has wider benefits than the learning and problem-solving they are developed for.

References

Lave, J. and Wenger, E. (1991) *Situated Learning: Legitimate Peripheral Participation*. Cambridge: Cambridge University Press.

Lewis, D. and Allan, B. (2005) *Virtual Learning Communities: A Guide for Practitioners*. Buckingham: Open University Press.

Wenger, E., McDermott, R. and Snyder, W. (2002) *Cultivating Communities of Practice*. Boston, MA: Harvard Business School Press.

Wilson, B. and Ryder, M. (1996) *Dynamic Learning Communities: An Alternative to Designed Instructional Systems*. Available at: http://carbon.cudenver.edu/~mryder/dlc.html (accessed 28 November 2006).

9 Professional issues in online learning

Introduction

In adult learning, students have considerable autonomy in relation to how they go about their studies. The ethos of e-learning supports the notion of autonomy because it allows for flexible approaches to time management and access to information. However, autonomy generally brings with it responsibilities and duties and this is true of adult, flexible learning approaches. Hence this chapter will discuss some of these responsibilities and duties.

It is quite difficult in health and social care to separate professional, legal and ethical issues because there is considerable cross-over between the three topics. This chapter will, therefore, seek to address the issues together rather than look at each of the three in isolation. Nonetheless it is important to consider what is meant by the three topic headings, both in general and in the context of this chapter first.

The word 'professional' is becoming increasingly difficult to define. It is now used as a blanket term to refer to what a person is employed as. Previously, it was a term used to refer to specific areas of employment that were seen to have the characteristics of a 'profession' rather than a 'job', areas such as medicine, the law or religion. From a health and social care perspective, and therefore from the perspective of this chapter, the term refers to the code of expected behaviour that governs all those employed in the field, whether they are deemed to be 'trained' or 'untrained', 'qualified' or 'unqualified'. The issues discussed have relevance to all workers within the health and social care field who are undertaking any online learning in relation to their role. The title of practitioner in this context also refers to anyone involved in the delivery of health and social care.

The difference between legal and ethical issues can be equally difficult to understand at times. However, legal in this context refers to those aspects of online learning that are governed by the law of the land. Within this chapter, the law is English law; however, many countries have a similar approach to the issues and Internet specific law tends to be international because of the global access. Ethical issues may be the same as legal issues but where the approach and guidance may differ somewhat. Ethics discusses 'rights' and 'wrongs' from a moral perspective rather than what is allowed or not allowed by law. For example, the law in the United Kingdom allows abortion in certain circumstances but some people would take the ethical view that abortion is 'wrong' despite this. Many issues in health and social care require consideration from both the legal and ethical perspective and that is equally true of learning-related subject matter online.

Confidentiality

It is vital that the confidentiality of patients and clients is protected at all times. It is a requirement of all those who work within health and social care that measures are taken to prevent any information about patients and clients from becoming known to anyone not entitled to it. This requirement is part of the conditions of service and therefore in the contract of all health and social care workers. For many it is also a significant part of their professional code of conduct, for example, the Nursing and Midwifery Council (2004) Code of Professional Conduct (see Box 9.1).

In the United Kingdom the right to confidentiality for an individual is also protected by the Data Protection Act 1998 (see Box 9.2). This Act specifically relates to data stored electronically and although not directly related to health and social care or indeed online learning it is entirely relevant as it underpins the confidentiality guidance provided by employers and the professional bodies. It also clearly highlights that there are particular issues when considering computer-based material.

It is clear that in written work no real names should ever be used for patients and clients and that, in addition, acknowledgement of this protection is made to ensure that readers know that any names used are fictitious only. Extensive guidance in respect of this is often provided by your educational institution; if you are not aware of any, you should check the website or with your tutor. Failure to comply with confidentiality guidance can result in a penalty being applied and you may lose marks, or possibly even fail. It is therefore vital that you familiarize yourself with the rules of your particular course or module to avoid errors. It is also necessary to gain the consent of patients and clients for information about them to be used in academic work such as case studies or critical incident analysis. To prevent inadvertent recognition of patients and clients details such as hospital or NHS Trust names should be omitted from written work, details such as dates and times should not be used and any specific personal history avoided.

One of the essential features of online learning is electronic discussion and sharing of information. The rules on confidentiality apply here also. Maintenance of complete confidentiality can be more complex in discussion between learners. Places of work are likely to be known to each other and just as with face-to-face conversation, it can be tempting to include details that could be construed as a breach of confidentiality. This must be avoided at all

Box 9.1

Confidentiality

Whatever, in connection with my professional practice, or not in connection with it, I see or hear, in the life of men, which ought not to be spoken of abroad, I will not divulge, as reckoning that all such should be kept secret.

(The Hippocratic Oath,
as cited by McHale and Gallagher 2003)

As a registered nurse, midwife or specialist community public health nurse, you must protect confidential information. . . .
    You must guard against breaches of confidentiality by protecting information from disclosure at all times.

(Nursing and Midwifery Council 2004)

As a social care worker, you must strive to establish and maintain the trust and confidence of service users and carers. This includes: Respecting confidential information and clearly explaining agency policies about confidentiality.

(General Social Care Council 2002)

Radiographers are ethically and legally obliged to protect the confidentiality and security of patient information acquired through their professional duties, except where there is a legal requirement to do otherwise.

(College of Radiographers 2004)

Box 9.2

Principles of the Data Protection Act 1998

'Personal data' should be processed fairly and lawfully.
Explicit consent is given for the processing of the data.
Data should only be obtained for one or more specified purpose.
Data should be accurate and contemporaneous.
Data should be disposed of when no longer necessary.

(Department for Constitutional Affairs 1998)

costs. While your fellow learners are also bound by the rules of confidentiality, your discussion may not be as secure as is ideal. Just as conversations can be overheard, those who should not have access can see online discussions, despite password protection and other measures educational institutions take to avoid unauthorized access. Anonymize the details of your discussion as much as you possibly can and apply the rules that guide your written work to your online discussion. These measures need not detract from the value of your interaction in any way, but they will help to protect patients and clients from breaches of confidentiality.

Maintaining confidentiality is an ethical principle as well as a professional and legal one. Patients and clients need to be able to trust their professional carers in order to divulge information relevant to their care. In order to provide holistic care, it is often essential that patients or clients provide us with some very personal details about their lives and relationships. They will not do this if they feel vulnerable to breaches of confidentiality or even sharing of information with other professionals without their permission. Care cannot do active good (beneficence) if all relevant information is not available nor can the practitioner be sure that no harm is done (non-malifice). Patients cannot exercise their autonomy adequately if they do not trust the practitioner not to breach their confidentiality.

It is not just patients and clients who have a right to confidentiality. Colleagues are also entitled to this. All interactions and written work should ensure that no one can be identified in any way. This is an important issue because it is easy to forget and use the names or specific role titles of colleagues in discussion. Even positive comments that refer to a person specifically are a breach of their confidentiality and, although this may seem extreme, it is essential that good practice be adopted at all times. Informal discussion within online learning is a particular area where this issue may be forgotten as it is natural to refer to a peer, your manager or a colleague from another profession at the very least by role title, just as you would in conversation. You do need to take care online, however, as it is a more permanent record of your comments (see Box 9.3).

Box 9.3

Good practice for maintaining confidentiality in online discussions

- Do not use patients' or clients' names.
- Do not use the names of colleagues or even your friends.
- Do not use specific personal details of anyone, including role titles.
- CHECK BEFORE YOU SUBMIT.

Respect for persons

From an online perspective, respect for individuals has two elements to it: first, respect for patients and clients, and second, respect for your fellow learners. Respect for patients and clients means that you should always take care not to discuss them in an inappropriate manner. This links with maintaining confidentiality but is also about not being judgemental. Respect for your fellow learners relates to your behaviour in discussion groups and any other online communication. It is important that communication of any nature conforms to social norms and does not use inappropriate language, or include discriminatory or inflammatory comments.

It is an important part of e-learning that students interact and communicate in a way that is as near to face-to-face as is possible online. To achieve this, there is an element of informality in some activities and discussion forums. However, while this informality exists to encourage participation some caution does need to be exercised. Face-to-face interaction has the benefit of non-verbal communication that can make it clear that a joke is being made or a comment is not intended to offend. This is not always possible online. We often use phrases that are discriminatory without realizing it but care needs to be taken with this online. There is often the temptation to use electronic media to exchange jokes and, while it is important that learners have fun, it is also vital that offence is not caused.

Another aspect of demonstrating respect for your fellow learners is to allow for the fact that they might not have the same views as you. Discussion and debate within health and social care education is essential and a questioning approach to practice is healthy. Nevertheless debate should not become heated argument, particularly in a distance learning environment where discussion can become stifled by the anxiety caused by lack of tolerance or narrow-mindedness of the minority. In a classroom, such argument can be 'refereed' by the teacher and other learners but the time lag in electronic 'conversation' can be such that the damage is done before this can occur. It is also good practice for all health and social care practitioners to exercise control when discussing and debating practice because it is inappropriate to enter into heated argument with or in front of patients and clients. The advantage of online debate is that you have time to think while typing your response and therefore have time to apply a reasoned response rather than the impulsive one you may be tempted to use face-to-face.

Inappropriate language and discussion is not only about being abusive or discriminatory. One of the advantages of online learning is that it can allow a range of different health and social care practitioners to be taught together because of the flexibility of time and place. The flexibility also allows it to be used for international students. This does mean that students have to be careful not to use jargon-laden language that may exclude others from the debate. It is good academic practice to compose your comments and arguments in such a way that someone can understand them with very little knowledge of the subject matter and interprofessional and international learning provides an opportunity to develop this skill. It is also good practice to be able to give information clearly and concisely to colleagues, patients and clients in a manner that is understood (see Box 9.4).

Plagiarism

Plagiarism is a form of cheating that involves using someone else's work and passing it off as your own. It is a serious issue in academic work generally but is also particularly serious in relation to health and social care practitioners as it constitutes deceit and thereby breaches the trust the public have in all who work within the sector. Plagiarism takes two main forms: failure to reference sources of information and the copying of another's academic work. The latter is necessarily deliberate as copying significant sections or the whole of someone else's work is not done by mistake. Failure to reference may be inadvertent rather than deliberate but is nonetheless something that is taken seriously.

Plagiarism is taken very seriously because summative assignments are meant to test your knowledge and, particularly in health and social care, may lead to an academic award that results in promotion, greater responsibility or a registered qualification with a professional body. Some professional bodies, for example the Nursing and Midwifery Council, may consider some cases of plagiarism to be so serious as to be construed as professional misconduct. It could also be argued that where promotion and therefore an increase of pay is involved, acts of plagiarism could be construed as fraud. This is an extreme view of plagiarism but it does clearly highlight how serious it can be from both a professional and legal perspective.

Referencing your academic work avoids any accusation of cheating and it is basic academic courtesy to acknowledge the source of your information. Great care should be taken to ensure all sources of information are referenced

---

Box 9.4

Respect for individuals

Rule 4 – Relationships with professional staff and carers: Chartered physiotherapists shall communicate and cooperate with professional staff and other carers in the interests, and with the consent of their patient; and shall avoid inappropriate criticism of any of them.

(Chartered Society of Physiotherapy 2002)

6.5 Working openly and co-operatively with colleagues and treating them with respect.

(General Social Care Council 2002)

appropriately and guidance on the method required for your particular programme or module will be provided by the institution involved. However, referencing is central to all assignments and is by no means unique to e-learning. Online learning does encourage electronic searching and use of the Internet as a source of information though. This can lead to confusion with referencing but it can also provide access to material that can lead a student into the temptation to cheat. A wide range of material is available for sale online that is aimed at students. It is allegedly there to help with academic work but is also aimed at those who may wish to purchase work that they can then submit as their own. Do not be tempted! Academic markers are well aware that these materials are available and are often more aware of their students' abilities than they are given credit for. They can, therefore, spot inconsistencies of style or use of literature which is not readily available to their students. In addition, there are an increasing number of software packages available to screen for plagiarism.

Plagiarism is cheating and breaches the trust placed in students by their teachers, colleagues, managers and patients/clients. However, more importantly perhaps, students who commit plagiarism are cheating themselves. There is a great deal of satisfaction and a sense of self-worth to be gained from achieving success in assessment strategies. Health and social care education at any level is aimed at providing the knowledge and skills required to practice safely and competently, whether this is directly by clinically orientated education or indirectly by providing the ability to think and make decisions in a more effective, evidence based manner. Cheating means that you miss out on gaining the necessary skills and knowledge and that may leave you open to both professional and contractual discipline and/or legal action. At the very least, it may make your working life much more difficult as you struggle to perform without the relevant skills and knowledge. A lack of knowledge and skills in health and social care can leave patients and clients at risk particularly as it becomes difficult to admit the deficit (see Box 9.5).

Box 9.5

Avoiding plagiarism

- Always acknowledge the source of your information, both in the text of your work and in a reference list at the end using an appropriate referencing method.
- Avoid the use of direct quotes.
- When working together on a piece of work ensure that you do not write together or share written work that may then lead to distinct similarities between your assignments.
- NEVER COPY SOMEONE ELSE'S MATERIAL.

Intellectual property

Intellectual property rights refer to the rights of the person who designs the material for your online learning. Intellectual property rights have always existed in relation to traditional modes of learning; however, they are perhaps more complex in online courses where ownership of the material is less clear (Gilchrist and Ward 2006). From a student's perspective, though, the issues have greater clarity. The material provided online is for the use of students who have signed up to undertake the course or module and should not be shared with others not undertaking study in this context. Most online learning is performed in a password-protected environment to assist with protecting intellectual property rights. Your password should not be shared with anyone else and handouts should not be copied for your colleagues or friends. This is both a legal and ethical aspect of e-learning as while copyright law offers some protection in relation to intellectual property, there is also an issue of trust and honesty between learners and teachers.

You should not use the material provided to you by your online facilitators in your own teaching unless you have obtained explicit permission from the author. This is particularly important if the presentation or teaching session is part of an academic assessment, but consent must also be sought if the material is to be used for teaching students, patients, clients or colleagues.

Netiquette

Netiquette is a new word to address the matter of Internet etiquette; it is a catch-all term for electronic politeness. Netiquette is effectively a set of rules for appropriate online behaviour. Much of the above relates to netiquette but has been addressed separately because of the particular importance of the issues either to online learning, to health and social care practitioners or both. A central concept of netiquette is 'remember the human' (Shea 1990). It is easy to forget that there are people at the receiving end of your electronic discussion, particularly when you are part of a big group who did not previously have any social contact. Because of this, it is easier to forget the normal social conventions which govern our interactions and conversations. Shea (1990) offers a strong message that normal standards of behaviour apply to cyberspace as well as to life in general.

Rule 4 of Shea's (1990) netiquette relates to respecting other people's time and suggests that you should think carefully before sending a message or deciding who you copy into the message. If your work involves the use of email, you will be able to relate to this element of netiquette because there seems to be an ever greater reliance on electronic communication in the workplace and this, in turn, can attract 'spam' unless the security of your system is extremely good. There is however a balance to be had in relation to online learning. This mode of learning relies on the electronic interaction of the student group and so the discussion and debate within the discussion forums and the more social interactions between students are vital to the learning experience. For example, just because you are online at midnight, it does not mean that anyone else will be and you will need to wait for responses to your question, discussion point or comments. The main benefit of online learning lies in its inherent flexibility and learners will access discussion at different times and on different days as they fit their learning around their working and social life. This can lead to frustration as you wait for someone to respond to a discussion point or comment that you have made. Rest assured you will get a response; it may just take a little time. Shea (1990) also discusses sharing knowledge online. This is an aspect that is central to online learning, and indeed to learning in health and social care in general. There are often as many benefits from the sharing of knowledge and information between students as there are from the formal teaching. One of the advantages that is cited in relation to classroom teaching is the opportunity to network and discuss mutual interests with fellow learners in breaks from teaching. This is also possible online and sharing knowledge is very much a part of this. It does not matter whether it is professional knowledge or recipes or a critique of the latest film, it all helps to create a sense of community and therefore enhances the more formalized discussion. Finally, be tolerant of others' mistakes; we have all at some point made errors of judgement or typing and no doubt will again and we should understand that our colleagues will too (see Box 9.6).

Accountability

Accountability is generally thought of in health and social care as a professional issue; however, all health care professionals are legally accountable as well as professionally accountable for their actions, as illustrated in Box 9.7.

These arenas of accountability apply to learning as well as in practice. This chapter has addressed issues that the umbrella of accountability covers. All health and social care employees have a level of accountability within their role whether they are qualified or unqualified. Accountability is simply being able to answer and account for our actions and the difference generally between qualified and unqualified staff is the element of professional accountability and its relationship with professional misconduct. In online

---

Box 9.6

Netiquette: the basic rules

- Be polite.
- Be tolerant.
- THINK BEFORE YOU SUBMIT!

Box 9.7

Arenas of accountability

Professional
To the professional body (e.g. Nursing and Midwifery Council, General Medical Council, Health Professional Council). This relates to professional misconduct and professional regulation to protect patients or clients and their families.

Employer
Through employment law and contracts of employment, the health care professional is accountable to their employer to adhere to conditions of service and corporate policies or guidelines.

Public
Through civil law, health care professionals can be held to account for their actions and to pay compensation where appropriate.

Criminal
There is now a raised awareness that some health care professionals may need to be called to account in criminal courts not only for obvious criminal acts (murder, manslaughter, rape, theft) but also for criminal negligence.

(Dimond 2005)

---

learning, each and every person contributing to the experience needs to consider their accountability in relation to each other as previously discussed in this chapter. Clearly, issues such as confidentiality and gaining consent for inclusion of clinical information about patients or clients come under the heading of professional accountability. This has been highlighted by reference to the Codes of Conduct and Standards of Practice of the various bodies associated with professional regulation in health and social care. It is also a requirement for most practitioners to maintain their knowledge and skills, and this underpins not only the learning undertaken in general terms but also the need to ensure that you access literature and research that is current and valid to support your learning.

There is also the question of accountability to your employers if the course or module is being paid for and/or study time is being provided. Support from your employer is a valuable asset and should not be abused by not putting in appropriate effort to your studying. Accountability in this respect also requires learning to be put into practice rather than simply used to enhance your own curriculum vitae or promotion prospects. Employers who are paying for their employees' professional development do so from a perspective of self-interest. They do so to improve the overall quality of the service they provide. Equally, however, you have a responsibility to highlight any difficulties you experience to your managers if the promised support is not available to you or is not sufficient for you to gain from the experience. Remember that the priority always has to be care of patients and clients, and managers may need to amend their commitment to professional development for staff in response to staff shortages.

Accountability to the public in relation to learning revolves around the notion that personal professional development should be reflected in improved patient or client care. It is therefore incumbent on the learner to ensure that they undertake programmes of study that are relevant to their role and that the knowledge and skills gained are taken back into practice to develop the evidence base of care. This also ensures that clinical governance is being adhered to in respect of evidence-based practice.

An important aspect of evidence-based practice that can be actively improved by means of online learning is knowledge of relevant quality Internet information that may be helpful to patients/clients and their families. Increasingly patients/clients are aware of the wealth of information available to them and they wish to learn more about their condition and treatment for themselves. The Internet is a source of information that patients/clients often turn to and it is vital that they are provided with guidance as to which sites are relevant and provide evidence-based material, and which sites provide unsound advice and guidance or are not relevant to the health system they are being cared for within. Online learning encourages access to web-based material and offers the opportunity to explore what is available, thereby giving the learner insight into suitable sites for their client group. This information can then be shared with patients/clients and their families ensuring that they have the opportunity to improve their knowledge of their condition and treatment in an appropriate way. Arguably, provision of this type of information is an essential part of maintaining accountability to patients/clients and their families. Guidance in respect of online sources has been provided for you in Chapter 5 and you can use the skills identified there to enhance the information you provide for your patients/clients and their families. You can use it to inform your own interactions with them and you can provide them with appropriate web addresses within any written information you give them to support your verbal communication. This sharing of information clearly links with your accountability to the public.

The notion of criminal accountability has very limited applicability to learning online, or indeed learning by any means. However, there is one clear issue that is particularly pertinent to e-learning and that is access to inappropriate and unlawful Internet sites. There has been much media coverage of the problems of Internet pornography, particularly in relation to paedophilia. The difficulty for learners of health and social care is that it is sometimes possible to undertake a perfectly innocent search for a topic and find you have accessed a site that has nothing to do with health and social care.

If you have concerns about a site you have accessed being unlawful, you should inform someone about this. This is particularly important if you are using a computer at work or in a library because your inappropriate hit may be noted and will be traceable to you. Failure to report it may lead others to believe that access to the site was not an accident. The safest action you can take in relation to this is to be very careful about your selection of search terms and even more careful about opening unfamiliar sites.

Conclusion

This chapter has highlighted the major professional issues relating to online learning in health and social care. Many of the issues will be familiar to you in relation to practice but not perhaps in respect of your learning. Most of the issues, for example confidentiality and plagiarism, are pertinent to all aspects of learning, not just online learning. All the issues however have particular relevance to e-learning and this chapter should have provided you with some guidance for maintaining your professional integrity while enjoying the flexibility of online learning.

Netiquette has been discussed and is fundamental to your learning experience. From an ethical perspective, it is important to behave online in such a way as to avoid offending your fellow learners and your tutor. While the rules of netiquette are not specific to health and social care, they can be readily applied. Knowledge of the code of conduct or standards of practice, where applicable, is as essential to your learning as it is to your practice. Similarly, you need to be mindful of your underlying commitment to your patients/clients and your employer in relation to using your learning to maintain and improve the quality of care you provide. Online learning should be an enjoyable experience and the basic rules should ensure that all involved do gain maximum benefit from it. The main rule must be however:

THINK BEFORE YOU SUBMIT!

References

Chartered Society of Physiotherapy (2002) *Rules of Conduct*. Available online at: http://www.csp.org.uk/director/effectivepractice/rulesofconduct.cfm (accessed 28 November 2006).

College of Radiographers (2004) *Statements for Professional Conduct*. London: College of Radiographers. Available online as a PDF file at: http://www.sor.org/public/pdf/profcond2.pdf (accessed 24 August 2006).

Department for Constitutional Affairs (1998) *Data Protection Act*. Available in full online at: http://www.opsi.gov.uk/ACTS/acts1998/19980029.htm (accessed 24 August 2006).

Dimond, B. (2005) *Legal Aspects of Nursing*, 4th edition. Harlow: Pearson Longman.

General Social Care Council (GSCC) (2002) *Codes of Practice for Social Care Workers and Employers*. London: GSCC. Available online at: http://www.gscc.org.uk/Home/ (accessed 24 August 2006).

Gilchrist, M. and Ward, R. (2006) Facilitating access to online learning. In: Glenn, S. and Moule, P. (eds) *E-learning in Nursing*. Chapter 6. Basingstoke: Palgrave.

McHale, J. and Gallagher, A. (2003) *Nursing and Human Rights*. Edinburgh: Butterworth Heinemann.

Nursing and Midwifery Council (NMC) (2004) *The NMC Code of Professional Conduct: Standards for Conduct, Performance and Ethics*. London: NMC. Available online at: http://www.nmc-uk.org/aFramedisplay.aspx?documentID=201 (accessed 24 August 2006).

Shea, V. (1990) *Netiquette*. Available online at: http://www.albion.com/netiquette/ (accessed 24 August 2006).

10 Clinical and communication skills and online learning

Introduction

In the context of this chapter, the phrase 'clinical skills' will refer to any practical skill necessary to perform the role of a health and social care practitioner. It will therefore include those skills needed to carry out social care as well as those more commonly associated with health care delivery. Health and social care is essentially skills based, although it is also necessary for practitioners to carry out skills knowledgeably. Clinical and communication skills are central to learning for practice whether as a novice or as part of professional development. Decision-making is also part of all practitioners' roles, whether qualified or unqualified. At the very least, a minimum level of decision-making relates to the need to refer to someone else, and the range then goes through a continuum to making a diagnosis, whether this is medical or professional in a different context. Online learning can offer a wide range of facilities to allow you to develop your skills as well as your knowledge.

Learning skills

There is a widely held belief that skills can be learned only by doing (experiential learning) and this can take place only in laboratories or classrooms and actual workplace situations with careful supervision by a teacher with the relevant skills. This belief is being challenged by new ways of learning and a distinct shift away from the traditional pedagogical methods of teaching to a more student-led and problem-solving approach to learning. There are now a range of means available to simulate situations and allow students to learn in a safer way than the 'trial and error' of an apprentice-type training. This also allows them to gain a deeper understanding of not just how to do something, but why they are doing it. It is generally accepted that the 'sit with Nellie' or 'see one, do one' approaches to gaining job-related skills do not constitute good quality teaching or result in high quality care provision. This is true of all education and training in health and social care, but is particularly relevant to online learning where teachers have had to be innovative in providing knowledge and skills in relation to the practicalities of doing the job.

Educational theory clearly highlights that the essence of learning a skill is to be able to learn the elements of the task by being taught and seeing a demonstration and then perfecting your own technique by carrying it out under supervision (Curzon 1990). Theorists differ on their view of how this actually occurs but fundamentally agree on the main principles. Traditionally this has taken place by means of a taught demonstration followed by practice, either in a laboratory or classroom setting or in the practice setting. Most nurses, for example, can remember learning how to do an intramuscular injection and the first one they actually gave to a patient. Some skills, and injection is perhaps an example, are still arguably best learned in this way, particularly since manikins and other similar equipment are now available and allow practice to be as near real as possible without a patient being subjected to the very first attempt. However, not all skills have to be learned in this way. Health and social care is wide and varied in the skills required and different techniques can be applied to learning how to deliver patient or client care.

Skills in health and social care are not purely motor skills in perhaps the same way as manual workers demonstrate their ability to do the job. Practitioners need to have the ability to communicate, assess, plan and implement a range of interventions depending on patient/client need, the circumstances and their role. Online learning techniques can be influential in gaining skill in care, and are perhaps in some cases ideally suited to assisting practitioners develop their practice to a high level.

Online videos

Demonstration of a skill is very much a part of the learning and teaching process. It is essential that as the learner you see how something is done both as a whole and in the constituent parts of the task. As already highlighted, this has traditionally been done by a classroom or laboratory-based teaching session to a single learner or small group with either a volunteer 'patient/client' or a manikin or in practice with a real patient or client. As discussed briefly in Chapter 7, online learning allows the use of video clips of the skills demonstration. This allows you to watch the demonstration as many times as you like and also to return to it having practised for yourself. In many ways, this method of skills teaching has advantages over a classroom or practice-based learning because you can learn at your own pace and you have a good view of the demonstration for there is no one else to impede it. It is necessary, though, to have access to a computer that has the software and speakers to allow you to hear the commentary.

The demonstrations can be embedded into the virtual learning environment or they can be packaged in a separate DVD. They have the distinct advantage that you can rewind or fast forward to the particular aspect you wish to. This is particularly useful for more complex skills but may be just as useful for the novice learning the basics for the first time (see Figure 10.1).

This type of skills teaching can be used for a wide range of practice skills, from simple tasks such as hand washing to more complex aspects of care such as treatments, examinations and communication skills. The videos may relate to simulated events or may be, in some cases, films of actual interventions used with the express permission of the patient or client. The demonstration provided can be linked to activities and discussions for you to link theory to practice. The demonstration or scenario provided can be linked to a discussion thread that encourages you to discuss and debate the various elements of the skill involved.

Virtual patients or clients

One way of learning knowledge and skills relating to practice is using virtual patients (see Figure 10.2). This allows tutors to create scenarios involving patients or clients with a particular problem or set of problems which students can then work either individually or in groups to address. Some of the approaches to this are described in Chapter 7. In many ways, this is very much

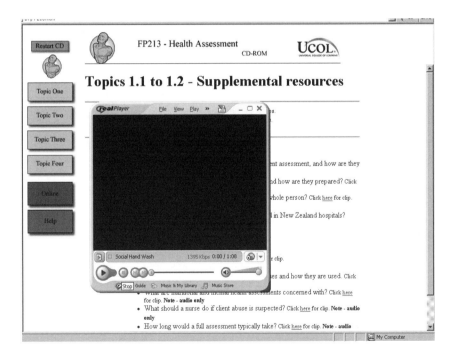

Figure 10.1 Example of a video clip supporting a CD-Rom package

(Reproduced with kind permission from Wendy Day, University College of Learning New Zealand)

Address:	http://..........	
	Courses> Critical Care of the Newborn>Scenarios	
	92379: Critical Care of the Newborn	
Course Menu Announcements Course Information Learning Resources Web Links Discussion Boards Chat Room Email Tools Help		**Scenarios**
		Monday 6th November 2006 **Peter**
		You are about to admit Peter a 26-week gestation baby who was born by caesarean section following a marked exacerbation of his mother's pregnancy induced hypertension. Peter is markedly growth retarded and needed resuscitation at birth (Apgars 2@1; 6@5). He is currently intubated and ventilated using 40% oxygen. What are your immediate nursing priorities? What are Peter's potential problems in the next 24 hours and what can you do to avoid or minimise these? Use the 'Peter' discussion board to discuss your thoughts on his care needs.

Figure 10.2 Example of a patient-based scenario for discussion

the same as much of the group work used in the traditional classroom; however, the advantage of online learning is that the information can be available for longer and tutors can build on the scenario or provide feedback as you work on it.

The virtual patient in Figure 10.2 represents a scenario for a group of nurses undertaking a course relating to their specialism of Special and Intensive Care of the Newborn. This scenario can be built on as the module progresses and you can then not only learn how to manage the baby's care but also see how babies like Peter progress or deteriorate as they would in real life (Figure 10.3).

As tutors, we can amend scenarios like Peter's according to your responses and introduce new situations that will impact on the care plan in different ways. This helps to replicate, as closely as possible, real situations where the patient's or client's needs and problems are often complex and one problem can have an effect on another. Figure 10.4 demonstrates how Peter has progressed to a new stage in his care. You can also have access to other people's responses as they work to provide care solutions for the virtual patient or client in a much more concrete way than is sometimes available in the classroom. This is particularly useful in post-qualifying programmes or modules where different approaches may be taken due to different local

Address:	http://..........	
	Courses> Critical Care of the Newborn>Discussion Boards	
	92379: Critical Care of the Newborn	
Course Menu		**Peter**
Announcements		I think the nursing priorities are immediate baseline observations. He will need Oxygen saturation monitoring, cardiac monitor, respiratory rate, temperature and blood glucose. Kate
Course Information		
Learning Resources		
Web Links		
Discussion Boards		
Chat Room		
Email		I agree Kate. It will also be important to take a photo for Mum, as she won't be able to visit. Jo
Tools		
Help		
		Blood gases might be useful too. Dave
		I think blood gases are not an immediate priority Dave as it would be better to allow Peter to settle first otherwise they will not provide an accurate picture of his condition overall. Liz (Tutor)

Figure 10.3 Example of a student response to a case study discussion

policies or different levels of experience. Use of the discussion boards in this context allows the students to ask questions and debate points made and this is essential for learning about practice. This point has been made elsewhere in this book and is central to online learning generally. It is particularly essential in these types of situation because discussion and debate here encourages the questioning of practice and thereby enhances the evidence base and the quality of care provision.

Virtual patients lend themselves to enhancing recognition of inter-professional working. Groups of students from different professional backgrounds can work together on a virtual patient or client scenario and discuss their differing priorities and approaches. This in turn can lead to a greater understanding of different practitioners' roles in care provision and better management of care in practice. Interprofessional learning and interprofessional working are both high on the health and social care agenda currently as there is a growing recognition that practitioners need to be able to work together to provide seamless care which is both evidence based and costeffective. Patient or client expectations are high and their needs are often complex. In the past, care provision has been lacking in communication, which can result in replication and conflicting information. Working together on virtual patient or client scenarios can improve this situation and create better working relationships, which then have a positive impact on care provision.

Address:	http://..........	
	Courses> Critical Care of the Newborn>Scenarios	
	92379: Critical Care of the Newborn	
Course Menu		Scenarios
Announcements		**Monday 13th November 2006**
Course Information		**Peter**
Learning Resources		Peter has now been in a cot for 24 hours.
Web Links		However, his temperature last time you took it
Discussion Boards		was slightly high at 37.3 and is now 35.7. There is
Chat Room		no obvious environmental reason for this drop in
Email		temperature. He had a small vomit after his last
Tools		feed and he is less responsive to handling when
Help		you give his 'cares'.
		What are the possible causes of Peter's
		observations?
		What can you do to determine the actual cause?

Figure 10.4 Example of a progressing case scenario

Working together can be an element of the module being studied as in the example in Figure 10.5 or can be as a result of the same scenario being shared between different students studying the same subject matter using the same discussion forums.

The Jessica scenario is to encourage a mixed group of learners to offer their own solutions to the issues raised by her situation. Their thoughts can then be shared on the discussion board and each member of the group can then discuss them and/or ask questions.

For this type of interprofessional learning to work, all members of the group must be committed to socializing and contributing to the discussion and debate. As before, Jessica's scenario can be developed and her case followed to allow learners to apply theory to practice and discuss differing professional approaches to her care and support. This discussion and debate can potentially be more in-depth and detailed than in a classroom setting, allowing learners to gain insight into what can be done for clients with complex health and social care needs.

Similarly, practitioners can gain insight into cultural aspects of care, particularly where international learners are involved. Jessica's scenario could be changed to that of a woman from any country in the world, situated in either her home country or an adopted one, to encourage learners to consider cultural aspects of care and the differences in care and services in other communities.

Either of the two virtual patients/clients detailed here could also be linked to video clips demonstrating particular skills related to their care. These can be health care skills such as attaching a transcutaneous oxygen monitor to

Address:	http://..........	
	Courses>Interprofessional Approaches to Working with Older People >Scenarios	
	97789 Interprofessional Approaches to Working with Older People	
Course Menu		**Scenarios**
Announcements		**Thursday 9th November 2006**
Course Information		**Jessica**
Learning Resources		Jessica is 78 years old. She currently lives alone in a council flat in an inner city area. The flat is on the fourth floor and the lift works only intermittently. Recently Jessica has developed bilateral leg ulcers and finds walking any distance difficult. She has meals on wheels twice a week but is not eating much in between these. She is however fiercely independent and is reluctant to accept any assistance from professional carers.
Web Links		
Discussion Boards		
Chat Room		
Email		
Tools		
Help		
		What do you consider are Jessica's immediate care needs and who do you think should provide them?

Figure 10.5 Example of an online discussion scenario designed to facilitate interprofessional collaborative communication using a client scenario and online discussion

Peter or assessing Jessica's leg ulcers, or broader skills, such as approaches to discussing Peter's care with his parents or a case conference in relation to Jessica's care needs.

Virtual hospitals

A logical progression from virtual patients is the virtual hospital, where scenarios are linked not only to individual patients, but also to the facilities available and the difficulties encountered in the 'real world' of health care where there is a lack of resources, beds and facilities (Sharp and Primrose 2003). This takes the notion of closing the theory–practice gap still further and encourages you to be resourceful in providing high quality care within the constraints of a less than perfect service. It also can be used to help with prioritizing within a virtual ward or department.

Virtual hospitals can be used to teach patient care from a range of perspectives; they are also useful areas where different students can have shared access and learn from learners from different professional backgrounds and different levels of experience. The virtual hospital can be used for a wider variety of skills, not only the direct care of patients but also management and leadership, resource management and estates management.

Virtual communities

Taking this concept a step further is the development of a virtual community. A virtual community, usually a website with the features of a community laid out in it, can be an area of a town or city to provide insight into, for instance, a socially deprived community. It can also be a whole town that provides an array of different situations from a wide range of financial and cultural backgrounds. This approach can provide a wealth of practice situations for learners and encourage the link between primary and secondary care, and between health care and social care.

The virtual community allows you to consider the patient or client in their own environment and see how relationships, social background, culture and education all impact on care needs. Visual details can be provided and demographic information enhances the virtual reality of a community with a range of individual and family issues which need health and social care input. The community, like the hospital, will have a particular range of facilities to support patient need. The interprofessional and international approaches to learning are further enhanced in the virtual community.

This can be widened from just health and social care to relationships with other people who play a part in the lives of patients and clients occasionally and impact on care needs and problems, such as police officers, local authority officers and the voluntary sector. You can be provided with a much wider scenario to allow you to enhance your understanding of the importance of communication and planning in relation to the care of an individual. The notion of a virtual community also encompasses the holistic approach to care that is central to health and social care philosophy.

Like the virtual hospital, the community can help teach wider skills such as management and leadership. A very important element of health and social care provision that can be addressed online by means of a virtual community is disaster management. This has become a vital aspect of preparation for staff across a wide range of services, as situations such as major incidents, terrorist attack and pandemic influenza have to be considered and practised. Preparing for these types of incidents, even if only in part, reduces the disruption they inevitably incur.

Communities of practice

These have been extensively discussed in Chapter 8, but have clear relevance to the learning of practice-based skills as the rationale for a community of practice is to address, collectively, a work-based issue or problem. An inevitable effect of this has to be that participants enhance their relative practice skills and knowledge. Communities of practice may also arise from the groups undertaking formal learning within an online module or programme as their discussion progresses to the point where it is clear that they have a mutual interest or problem that may be best served by this particular online approach.

Communication skills

One issue that has been a constant problem within health and social care is that of communication. The majority of complaints relate to the lack or inadequacy of communication between practitioners. This is, therefore, a vital skill to learn. Online learning can be helpful in this respect, despite the lack of face-to-face interaction. Indeed, some learners would suggest that it is the lack of face-to-face interaction that makes the virtual learning environment suited to gaining confidence in communication. Online learning requires you to contribute to discussion and debate and generally socialize with the other students. Without this level of interaction, the value of your learning is limited. You should therefore be able to enhance your ability to communicate in writing by means of the discussion forums provided within your learning package.

This is not the only skill you should gain in respect of communication however. Within discussion and debate you should be learning how to make your point assertively and firmly without causing offence or being unduly aggressive. This is a skill that is most useful in your working life because being an advocate for your patients or clients involves the ability to be assertive without crossing the line into unprofessional and angry exchanges. The level of discussion and debate encouraged within online learning should enhance understanding of another point of view and an ability to question what you do not understand or are not sure of. The nature of the online learning environment allows you to make your point or ask your question without having to wait for a lull in discussion as can happen in face-to-face interaction. This alone can enhance your confidence in communicating your point in any situation, particularly if you gain positive feedback from your fellow learners.

Scenarios can be provided for you, by any of the means already discussed in this chapter, that directly encourage you to consider how to communicate in a given situation. Online learning provides you with the opportunity, should you chose to accept it, to think your responses through because an immediate response is not as essential as it can be in a classroom. This should encourage you to apply the theory you have learned into practice and consider good practice in relation to communicating in a given situation.

Communication skills relate to more than written or debating skills. There is also the very important aspect of being able to provide information in a way that patients or clients and their families can understand and utilize to make informed decisions about care and services. For example, in the case of the Special and Intensive Care of the Newborn course, a useful exercise for the students would be one similar to the example in Figure 10.6.

Address:	http://..........	
	Courses> Critical Care of the Newborn>Scenarios	
	92379: Critical Care of the Newborn	
Course Menu		Scenarios
Announcements		**Monday 4th December 2006**
Course Information		**Peter**
Learning Resources		Peter is progressing well however because of his
Web Links		prematurity he will need screening for retinopathy
Discussion Boards		of prematurity. You will need to gain informed
Chat Room		consent from his mother for this screening.
Email		
Tools		What do you think are the potential problems in
Help		gaining consent?
		What issues do you need to be sensitive about?

Figure 10.6 Example of an activity designed to facilitate discussion and debate about practice

The key issue raised in the scenario in Figure 10.6 is that students need to recognize that they will have to make it clear that Peter may have a significant visual impairment, hence the need for screening. For a mother whose infant has survived a difficult critical care stage and is now apparently progressing, possible bad news will not be easy to take in or accept. The balance between providing truthful information about the level of risk and reassurance is a difficult one, but online discussion about different experiences and ideas can enhance learning in a way that does not inflict 'trial and error' on actual patients or clients. Similarly, scenarios relating to social care situations such as child protection, dealing with dementia, and discussing financial issues can be used to enhance learning in a safe and supportive environment. Such scenarios can in addition be supported by videos of good practice.

Important communication issues such as imparting bad news and managing conflict can be discussed online. Good practice in communicating with special needs clients, children and those with hearing impairment can be shared and discussed in a virtual learning environment. The virtual patient, hospital or community can be useful here as scenarios can be developed and amended to represent the sort of problems and issues that would be experienced in practice.

The nature of online learning and the way it lends itself to interprofessional and transcultural exchanges that in turn improve understanding and communication in practice. Professional and cultural barriers can be a factor in problems and complaints relating to communication and it is important that the learning environment assists in reducing these. An example of the importance of learning to communicate across professional barriers can be found in child protection. Many reports have been issued regarding this over the years, such as in the United Kingdom, the Laming Report (2003) in respect of the death of Victoria Climbié. It essential that all health and social care professionals communicate effectively with each other and online learning can provide a learning environment that assists with this in a more flexible and interactive way than can sometimes be achieved in the classroom or in the pressures of the working environment.

Decision-making skills

Decision-making is central to the role of many health and social care workers. It has been thought of as the domain of medical staff and some senior practitioners in other professions, rather than something everybody does. However, as patient/client needs have become more complex and the demands on services have become greater, decision-making has become more important in a wide range of roles. Recognition of this has led to the inclusion of the subject in many teaching curricula. Online learning can also address the need to enhance decision-making skills.

We have already discussed the idea of virtual patients or clients and communities and how they can be used to learn clinical knowledge and skills. This has distinct links with developing decision-making skills – the patient/client scenarios provided either as individual cases or as part of a virtual hospital or community encourage you to think about assessing and planning care. This is very much about decision-making in a professional sense. The interprofessional learning already highlighted also enhances decision-making for a greater knowledge of the role of others in care provision will inform a more holistic approach to your decisions. The key element in decision-making is knowledge and information; learning should improve your knowledge and online learning can enhance your information gathering as you develop questioning skills and have access to the assessment and planning approaches of your fellow learners. A structured way of approaching a problem is seen as the central tenet of rational decision-making as described by Harbison (1991: 405): 'an analysis of the situation should be carried out, subsequent actions should be rational and logical, and the nurse should be able to make her knowledge and judgment explicit.' Harbison is referring to decision-making by nurses; however, this is applicable to any health and social care practitioner. Online learning by means of its interactive approach can encourage you to develop a more structured means of coming to a decision about the care of your patient/client (see Figure 10.7).

The scenario in Figure 10.7 encourages students to link the history obtained from the patient to the decision-making process related to diagnosis. The scenario can then be developed to include the rest of the assessment and examination of John. This will help you to identify and discuss the process with others undertaking the module. Feedback from your colleagues on the module and your tutor can then help you to refine your diagnostic reasoning.

Address:	http://..........	
	Courses> Minor Injuries>Scenarios	
	47576: Minor Injuries	
Course Menu		**Scenarios**
Announcements		**Thursday 26th October 2006**
Course Information		**John**
Learning Resources		John is 24 years old and has presented to the
Web Links		Minor Injuries Unit with an ankle injury.
Discussion Boards		
Chat Room		What information can you gain from a verbal
Email		history from John?
Tools		
Help		How will this information aid diagnosis?

Figure 10.7 Example of an assessment skills based scenario

The module used in the example is a nursing-focused one; however, such a module could be accessed by physiotherapists and radiographers who could offer a different perspective on the information gathering they would need to assist with their decision-making processes. Equally other interprofessional modules, such as child protection or care of the older person, could help with the different professional perspectives on assessment and decision-making.

It is possible to take this process further if the tutor adds detail to John's history, assessment and examination so that you can actually offer a diagnosis. This can be stressful for learners because they fear being wrong. The advantage of online learning, however, is that if you are really nervous about being incorrect, you can have one-to-one contact with your tutor until you gain confidence. This means of developing decision-making and diagnostic reasoning skills can therefore be better for those who find it difficult to voice an opinion in a group for fear of being wrong. It is helpful when you do get to use your skills in practice to have had the chance to try them out in the relative safety of a virtual learning environment. It is essential though that you do ultimately learn to offer an opinion to the rest of the group because the reality of practice is that you will have to be positive and assertive in relation to your decision in order to gain the confidence and trust of your patient or client and your colleagues. Again, online you are dealing only with hypothetical situations and if you are wrong, it is your pride that is hurt, not a patient or client. You will not have the face-to-face contact that makes being wrong particularly difficult either. The important thing to remember is there is always an element of trial and error in the learning process, and decision-making in health and social care is a complex skill.

The use of scenarios and feedback on clinical findings could be described as a virtual objective structured clinical examination (OSCE) which is a commonly used means of assessment for a range of health and social care practitioners. The development of your decision-making and diagnostic reasoning skills in this way can provide sound preparation for a summative OSCE, either in the module or programme you are undertaking online or in your future professional development. This means of teaching and learning also relates closely to the concept of problem-based learning.

As discussed briefly in Chapter 7, problem-based learning has been embraced by many health and social care professions as a means of developing skills that will enhance practice. It does this by preparing students in a meaningful manner for the reality and complexity of practice. Using scenarios is a central aspect of problem-based learning and therefore this online approach is entirely congruent with the current approach to health and social care education. The scenario can be linked with an online video to enhance the reality of the problem-solving process and this also is an aid to the OSCE assessment.

Development of decision-making skills requires some understanding of the process. A structured approach is central to ensure that you make the most of the information and time available to you to decide what you will do or what your diagnosis is. Diagnosis in this context need not be disease related as in medical practice but a means of determining patient or client need in a professional manner. There are models of decision-making offered by various authors and these are, for the most part, based on studies of the way practitioners make their decisions. You can apply these to your online learning as well as to actual practice to help you structure your thinking in a formal way, although you may develop your own process over time. The model detailed in Box 10.1 is based on diagnostic reasoning by doctors and offers a four-stage approach. You could use this in relation to your area of practice whether you are a health or social care practitioner.

The data collection element of decision-making can be applied to any situation because this is always central. You always need to gain information about the patient or client or the situation before considering your action. This can be achieved by history taking, assessment, examination or a combination

---

Box 10.1

Four-stage model of decision-making

1   Data collection.
2   Hypothesis generation: generating alternatives or options.
3   Cue interpretation: clarifying the evidence collected in the light of the hypotheses.
4   Hypothesis evaluation: reaching a judgement.

(Elstein et al. 1978)

of all of these. For example, if you are presented with a scenario involving an elderly woman needing social care provision, you would need in the first stage to assess her situation and her particular needs and problems. The second stage then relates to options available: what are the possible means of meeting the woman's needs? This may involve finding out more information about what services are available but if the scenario is set in a virtual community, you will have as much information as you would when you are fulfilling your working role. The third stage then requires you to clarify what may be the best of the options; in this case what she would prefer and what will best meet her particular requirements. In the fourth stage you would make a decision about the way forward and make this explicit to your tutor or on the discussion forum. Structuring your thinking in this way allows you to justify and be accountable for your decisions. Online learning allows some discussion about such decisions and this will help you not only to refine your skills but also to be able to be more assertive in relation to your chosen course of action or diagnosis.

An alternative seven-stage model in Box 10.2 is offered by Carroll and Johnson (1990). This builds on Elstein et al.'s (1978) four-stage model and reminds you that gaining feedback on your decision is an important element of the process. In online learning this will occur via your tutor and your student colleagues and provides you with vital insight into your decision. This also links with reflective practice, which clearly assists with honing your decision-making skills, particularly in relation to influencing factors such as stereotyping, assumptions and knowledge base.

Learning online with virtual patients or clients can provide you with the opportunity to confront preconceived ideas and assumptions without the trauma of making a less than effective decision in relation to a real situation.

Box 10.2

Seven-stage model of decision-making

1   Recognition: that a problem exists which requires a decision to be made.
2   Formulation: definition of the problem.
3   Alternative generation.
4   Information search.
5   Judgement or choice.
6   Action.
7   Feedback.

(Carroll and Johnson 1990)

In addition to the scenarios and virtual patients/clients you are presented with as part of the formal learning process, you can also discuss your practice experiences with your online colleagues as long as you maintain the confidentiality of all involved (see Chapter 9). Indeed you can set up a community of practice to guide your decision-making skills and assist with the implementation of evidence-based practice (see Chapter 8).

Learning and teaching skills

Though not strictly a clinical skill, teaching is very much a part of many health and social care practitioners' roles. There is a growing interest in e-learning as a means of providing statutory training, such as fire procedures and even resuscitation updates (Peterson 2006). Gaining skills in academic programmes is therefore a useful preparation for this type of in-service training.

It is also possible to gain knowledge and skills in facilitating learning by studying an online programme. This is going to be an increasingly useful skill as more and more training is by means of e-learning and as more technological means of supporting and assessing patients or clients are developed. Already there are telemedicine developments to support patients who require care from clinical teams at a distant centre. In addition it was shown in Chapter 8 that online communities of practice have much to offer practitioners in relation to work-based problem-solving and sharing good practice.

Mentor support

An important element of many programmes designed to develop practitioners' skills is the support of a mentor in the workplace. Mentors facilitate, supervise and assess learners in practice and are an invaluable source of support and encouragement. In traditional approaches to learning in health and social care, mentors have only limited access to the input students get from the educational institution. Online learning can however offer the mentor the opportunity to actively participate in formal learning activities and give them access to contact with the tutor to clarify any issues pertinent to their role. There are inevitably some difficulties with access to virtual learning environments but the benefits for all concerned are worth the effort.

Conclusion

This chapter has considered how online learning can enhance practical skills and knowledge as well as theoretical ones. Clinical and communication skills are central to high quality health and social care and as such have to be a major element of any education aimed at practitioners in the field. Online learning can offer the practitioner a wide range of activities to enhance their skills and aid decision-making in practice. This can be achieved by a variety of means and these can be employed either singly or in combination. Online learning can provide a viable forum for developing practice-based skills and knowledge that can enhance and support work based learning. The advantage of e-learning approaches to clinical skills is that your mentor can also have access to the teaching and learning materials, thereby having a clear picture of what is expected of you.

E-learning cannot replace hands-on work-based learning but it can offer a high quality means of safely gaining knowledge and skills that can be used in practice to care for patients or clients in an effective and caring manner.

References

Carroll, J.S. and Johnson, E.J. (1990) *Decision Research: A Field Guide.* London: Sage.

Curzon, L.B. (1990) *Teaching in Further Education: An Outline of Principles and Practice*, 4th edition. London: Cassell.

Elstein, A.S., Shulman, L.S. and Sprafka, A. (1978) *Medical Problem Solving: An Analysis of Clinical Reasoning.* Cambridge, MA: Harvard University Press.

Harbison, J. (1991) Clinical decision-making in nursing. *Journal of Advanced Nursing* 16 (44): 404–407.

Laming, Lord (2003) *The Victoria Climbie Inquiry.* London: HMSO.

Peterson, R. (2006) Teaching cardiopulmonary resuscitation via the Web. *Critical Care Nurse* 26 (3): 55–59.

Sharp, D.M. and Primrose, C.S. (2003) The 'virtual family': an evaluation of an innovative approach using problem-based learning to integrate curriculum themes in a nursing undergraduate programme. *Nurse Education Today* 23 (3): 219–225.

11 Assessment evaluation and research

Introduction

This chapter looks at the three issues of assessment, evaluation and research in relation to e-learning. It covers the construction and submission of assignments for e-learning assessment and provides practical advice around seeking support and guidance. The construction of academic work will be considered briefly. You can use the many books and websites focusing on study skills and assessment skills to provide you with deeper advice on, for example, writing essays. The aim of this chapter is to provide you with an overview and help you to get started. We must also consider both the evaluation of e-learning and research into online working since, as a student in a relatively new world, you are likely to be asked to give your opinions and reflections on the issues raised for you during the learning process.

Assessment

Assessment has several purposes. Traditionally, it is used to assess the amount and level of student learning achieved and to provide feedback on students' progress towards learning goals; in other words, it reports on progress and what has been achieved in terms of learning (Morgan and O'Reilly 1999: 15). Whatever the purpose of assessment, it should be generally used to demonstrate how a student has met the objectives or learning outcomes for a particular module of study. Essays and examinations have traditionally been the way that learning is assessed, especially so in health and social care. However, there is much debate about the value and reliability of these methods of assessment and, as e-learning develops, it is likely that new approaches to assessment may become a feature of courses. Providers of health and social care and educational institutions have been quite slow to adapt to the possibilities of online assessment in e-learning and blended learning programmes. As a consequence, many assessment modes in online learning are still traditional essays or examinations.

Assessment and the preparation for assessment are generally the most stressful aspects of any educational course or programme for most students. Let us begin by offering some tips for success and for reducing these stress levels: see Box 11.1.

Box 11.1

Tips for stress-free and successful assessment

1   Make sure that you understand what is being asked of you in terms of assessment right from the beginning of your course of study. Most course documents or handbooks will contain a description of the assessment. Some will provide quite detailed advice about how to go about the assessment. Whichever is the case, make sure that you use the section in your course or module guide on assessment as fully as you possibly can.

2   If you have any doubts or worries about the assessment, it is essential that you seek advice and ask questions of your tutor right from the outset, so that you are constantly improving your understanding of what is expected of you.

3   Note the deadline/s for the assessment submission and get started early. Many students leave commencing work on their assessment until the last minute. This is a stressful strategy that is practised with incredible regularity by students and is not the best way to learn. Tutors have little patience with students who leave their assessed work to the last minute – especially when other students successfully plan their time better.

4   When you start, make an action plan with dates for completing stages and try to stick to it.

5   Assume that everything you do in your online course contributes to your assessment and participate in it wholeheartedly. This will serve to make undertaking your assessment much more constructive and you will learn as you go along. You can return to archived discussion boards later to help with writing essays and other forms of assessment.

6   If you are writing a traditional essay or another form of written work and you have a choice of subjects to write about, try to make a decision about what you are going to write about early so that you can also start to search for the literature you need in plenty of time. This will lead to a much smoother approach to your assessed work.

7   If you are sitting an exam, try very hard to plan the study time you will need in order to learn or 'revise' what you need to pass the exam successfully. 'Cramming' a few days before the exam has always been a recipe for a stressful time and many students find it difficult to remember material they have tried to learn under pressure.

8   Do as much research as you can – using every resource possible.

9 Try to improve your writing and study skills by reading appropriate study skills books – some of these are identified in the further reading section of this chapter.

10 Constantly seek tutorial support from your tutor, either by email, discussion forum or chat room or even by telephone or face-to-face, if these are possible. Try asking your tutor if you can have regular small group tutorials in chat rooms or discussion boards on a regular basis to help you and other students get the idea of the assessment topics into your head. For many students in online and distance learning, the most substantial learning contact they have with their tutors is in feedback on their work (Simpson 2002: 44).

11 Make sure you have access to and understand how to operate any systems for handing in your written work, especially if this is to be submitted online.

12 If you receive feedback on your work from tutors, especially on formative work and on your assessed work, and you have not done as well as you would have liked, try to keep it in perspective and focus on finding out how you can do better next time.

Assessment of online learning

Assessment techniques have tended to lag behind innovation in online teaching methods (Maier and Warren 2000: 131). Some of this is because of the difficulty of preventing or recognizing cheating in online working. There are, however, many opportunities for the use of technology in assessment, both to make assessment more effective and to enhance learning. Computers can be used in a variety of ways to provide automatic feedback at important points in the learning process and can also be used for final (summative) assessment at the end of a course. This can involve individual students attending an assessment centre or may be conducted online, often using the college's virtual learning environment assessment systems.

One of the biggest problems with online learning assessment, for example when setting examinations online, is the ability to authenticate who has responded to the questions (Eaton and Moule 2006: 112). It is difficult to moderate the examination as you would do in a face-to-face situation, making sure that students do not cheat. These challenges are not totally insurmountable but involve educational institutions being more innovative in how they construct assessments. For example, it may be possible for students to sit what are known as 'seen' examinations online. Students are given the topic area, questions or subject of the examinations at some period of days, weeks or hours before the exam commences, but they write under examination conditions.

Online examinations and assessment tend to involve the following kinds of assessment (Maier and Warren 2000: 139; Clark 2004):

- multiple choice questions and other forms of online examinations
- self-assessment
- oral or online presentations or presentations using presentation software
- portfolios
- using spreadsheets and data processors to present information
- virtual experiments
- group work
- essays, reports and portfolios (word processed)
- multimedia essays using CD-Roms and websites.

You may come across some of these at various points in your online learning.

Discussion forum postings as assessment

One other likely option for online assessment is using student postings in discussion forums during the course of a programme or module to provide some form of continuous assessment of learning. Since the online discussion forums are so central in online learning, you may be informed from the outset that the discussions and group work that you produce online will be included as part of your assessment. The advantage of this is that the assessment event is not left until the end of the course. Your tutors should give you guidance, at the beginning of the course, to make sure that you understand what is expected of you in the discussion forums. Some say that assessment is said to shape-learning (Eaton and Moule 2006: 112), meaning that learning is enhanced and often driven by the assessment process. Being assessed as part of your online working is a form of continuous assessment and is a useful way of motivating students to participate in online discussions and shared work.

There are two central forms of assessment: formative and summative.

- **Formative assessment** is an approach that gives students the opportunity to submit work throughout the course of study. This enables tutors to give them feedback on their progress. Although feedback is given, it is not formally assessed and it does not count towards the final mark for the module or course. This approach is commonly used in open, distance and e-learning to motivate students to apply themselves to work throughout the course of study. In some cases formative assessment submission is compulsory and students will not be able to complete the final assessment unless they have submitted formative work for feedback.
- **Summative assessment** is generally conducted at the end of a course or module of study. This work is assessed and used in grading the student's achievements in that module of study.

Skills assessment

Away from the more traditional classroom methods, skills facility and practice setting based assessment of skill, the assessment of practical skills can be conducted in a variety of ways in the online environment. Computer simulation and OSCEs are just two ways that this might occur.

Objective structured clinical examinations (OSCEs) have become a common feature of assessment of health care practical skills and visual presentation of realistic situations is an important part of the process. Generated scenarios are presented at workstations, sometimes using role play or real or simulated patients or clients, with actors playing the part of the health or social care user (Eaton and Moule 2006: 113). Examples of using such strategies online are now starting to appear in the literature. Eaton and Moule (2006: 114) describe an OSCE examination used in the assessment of radiography students where the students' ability to assess and report on radiographic (X-ray) images is assessed online. It is important to note, however, that the examination took place in a computer room under examination conditions and the students did not take the examination from a distance.

Group working

In some online health and social care courses, the ability to work in a team or a group is an essential part of the achievement of the course outcomes. In order to assess this, your tutors may ask you to produce a piece of work as an online group or community. Many virtual learning environments will support this by enabling groups of students to work simultaneously on a document or number of documents, which they can share in an area of the VLE and create and edit as a group.

Working in groups is often no different online than face-to-face. It is fraught with relationship problems and group dynamics. For these reasons it is important that you set and agree ground rules as a group, especially if you are conducting a group piece of work for summative assessment. This way, those who have not made sufficient contribution to the work of the group can be challenged and supported.

Plagiarism

There is much debate about the need to move away from more traditional modes of assessment such as the essay or examination to improve the way we make judgements about student learning. Online working is a major feature of these issues. With the availability of such a mass of material online it is very easy for students to copy and paste large sections of text into their work, particularly written essays. Some students do this without acknowledging the original sources, possibly in an attempt to enhance the marks for their work.

This amounts to plagiarism, which is a form of cheating. Plagiarism is defined by Bassendowski and Salgado (2005: 1) as: 'the intentional or unintentional use of another's work or ideas, published or unpublished, without clearly acknowledging the original source of that work or idea'.

As discussed in Chapter 9, plagiarism is a professional issue as well as an academic one. In any educational setting it is not acceptable – and this is particularly so in health and social care education where ethics, altruism and morals are an integral part of practice. For these reasons, it is absolutely essential that, in written work of any kind, you acknowledge all of the sources of your ideas by referencing the material you have used correctly. It is, therefore, vital that you make sure you follow the referencing guidance of the educational institution with which you are working, for all of your written work, be it printed or online. All education providers now provide detailed guidance on how to avoid plagiarism and much of this will be offered in electronic format and online.

You should be aware that there are now computer programs which are designed to identify plagiarism in students' work. Tutors are able to use such programs to scan electronic copies of students' work to identify where they may have used the work of someone else without acknowledging it correctly. This is one of the many reasons why universities and colleges no longer accept hand-written work for assessment.

Submitting your work online

Even if your course or module uses a traditional essay approach to the assessment, many tutors will now ask for your work to be submitted online. The process for this will vary. Some tutors allow students to submit their work as an email attachment. However, there are also systems available within a VLE that enable you to submit your work into an online 'post box' system, sometimes known as a **drop box**. Some tutors may choose never to print out your work and use only the electronic document to read, assess and provide feedback from. If you are at all uncertain about how to use the online submission system used by your tutor, it is vital that you seek advice well before the hand-in deadline, so that you can submit your work on time.

In spite of the availability of online submission facilities, many tutors will still use more traditional approaches to hand-in of assessed work. If you are working from a distance you may be expected to hand your work in by normal postal delivery. It is important to check for certain what your education institution's guidance is on this. There will be deadlines for your work to arrive by and your tutor will have a system for logging the arrival of students' work. Many universities and colleges apply large penalties if work is late. For this reason, we would advise you to post your work early, especially if you are sending work to a tutor or institution in another country. There are often specific rules for overseas students in this respect. It is advisable that you ask for some kind of 'proof of posting' at the post office where you take your work to be mailed off. Some universities and colleges insist that posted work is sent by 'recorded' or some kind of 'special' delivery system. What is important, however, is that you can prove that you posted work on a certain date.

It probably goes without saying that it is absolutely *essential* that you keep at least one electronic copy and one hard paper copy of your work. Tutors will no longer accept excuses for the non- or late arrival of work because of computer problems. It is your responsibility to make certain that you have a back-up copy of your work that can be produced in an instant if your work has gone missing in transit. Tutors will be very suspicious of students who cannot produce a replacement for missing work immediately and your work may well automatically fail as a result.

Getting feedback

Feedback on your work will often take the form of written comments. Sometimes this feedback will be provided in the form of an electronic file. Microsoft Word® has a useful facility called 'Track Changes' and 'Comments' which allows your tutor, yourself and others to do two things:

1   Make the changes made to a document to be apparent to anyone reading the document. In order to do this, the system will highlight (often in red) changes as you go along when drafting, revising and editing work. Once the document is complete then you can accept the changes and the highlighting will disappear. This is particularly useful when work is being created by a group rather than just one individual.
2   Place comments within the text. These are generally highlighted in text boxes or bubbles in chosen places in the documents so that you can see clearly which section of your work a comment refers to. These can work in the same way as traditional comments that tutors might write on your written work in pencil or pen.

You may need to 'switch on' these facilities in the word processing program in order to use them. This option can generally be found in the Tools menu of Microsoft Word®. If you are unsure how to do this, or have problems, ask your tutor to talk you through it.

Evaluation

Student feedback of educational courses is essential. Teachers use such feedback to ensure that courses meet the needs of students. This is particularly important in online learning since the approach is still so new and educational institutions currently have little feedback on their successes and problems. Because of this, it is very likely that you will be asked to evaluate in relative depth online courses you undertake. Evaluation is concerned with gathering data and information to enable tutors and course designers to identify the outcomes and impact of the course or module and identify issues that need attention (Lewis and Allan 2005: 177).

There are a number of methods that your tutors are likely to use for evaluation purposes. However, it is most likely that you will be asked to fill in an evaluation questionnaire (either online or manually) which contains a number of closed and open questions about your experience of the course or module. Questionnaires can sometimes, but not always, be anonymized. You may also be asked to participate in an online discussion forum which is aimed at seeking your views and opinions – this is unlikely to be anonymous.

Whichever approach is used, your tutors will ask that you give a carefully thought out and honest opinion of your experience of the course. What they would also appreciate, however, is that you take a 'constructive' approach to your comments. There is a danger, when asked to evaluate a course, that students offer only the negative aspects of their experience. You should remember that your tutor is a human being and communicate your concerns about the course with regard for this. You should also try, as much as possible, to present the positive side of your experience.

Research

As e-learning is a relatively new method of education delivery it is possible that, as a student of an online course, you may be asked to participate in research into e-learning and the surrounding issues. There is currently a drive to research the value and effectiveness of e-learning across all education sectors. The existence of the 'E-learning Research Centre' (http://www.elrc.ac.uk, accessed 24 August 2006) bears witness to this in its aim 'to identify and investigate research problems in the field of e-learning that are of strategic importance for the sector as a whole'.

It is important to find out what impact e-learning has on students in terms of their learning, how this learning develops and what are the best ways of delivering learning online. To this end your tutors may well be undertaking some research to investigate these issues. As with all research studies, you must be asked for your consent to be involved in the research and you have every right to refuse if you wish. You may, for example, be asked to complete a questionnaire – either a paper or an online version. You should consider carefully whether you wish to participate in any research you are approached about and check out whether your responses are likely to be anonymized sufficiently for your responses to be unrecognizable by others in the final report (Eysenbach and Till 2000).

Online **focus groups** are one way that you may be asked to participate in research about online learning, for example, through analysis of your online discussion board postings. Using online discussion boards as 'virtual focus groups' is becoming quite a popular way of conducting research online (Moloney et al. 2003). Box 11.2 identifies some examples of the research

Box 11.2

Some examples of health and social care research related to online learning

Green, S.M., Voegeli, D., Harrison, M., Phillips, J., Knowles, J., Weaver, M. and Shephard, K. (2003) Evaluating the use of streaming video to support student learning in a first year life-sciences course for student nurses. *Nurse Education Today* 23 (4): 255–261.

Kenny, A.J. (2005) Interaction in cyberspace: an online focus group. *Journal of Advanced Nursing* 49 (4): 414–422.

Moule, P. (2006) E-learning for health care students – developing the communities of practice framework. (Includes radiography students). *Journal of Advanced Nursing* 54 (3): 370–380.

Rafferty, J. and Waldman, J. (2003) *Building E-learning Capacity for the Social Work Degree: A Scoping Study for the Department of Health E-learning Steering Group.* London: Department of Health.

studies that have been conducted into online working in health and social care. It is worthy of note that much of this research has been conducted in nursing education and that other health and social care disciplines still need to begin to develop a research base in this area.

Study and writing skills

Successful academic or practice assessment is often a product of your study and writing skills. Entire courses are provided and large numbers of books written on this subject and we strongly advise you to avail yourself of the benefit of these, especially if you are new to academic work or have not studied for some time. There are also a number of useful websites on these subjects and, once again, we recommend the Skills4Study website at www.skills4study.com as a good place to start.

Conclusion

Assessment is an important aspect of learning as well as a process of making judgements about student progress in online learning. Students need to think carefully about how they approach assessed written work and the range of other methods used in e-learning and blended approaches to learning.

Evaluation and research are important aspects of the development of online learning and the e-learning student has an important role to play in giving feedback to aid the future progress of this exciting way of learning.

References

Bassendowski, S.L. and Salgado, A.J. (2005) Is plagiarism creating an opportunity for the development of new assessment strategies? *International Journal of Nursing Education Scholarship* 2 (1) Article 3. Available at: www.bpress.com/ijnes (accessed 24 August 2006).

Clark, A. (2004) *E-learning Skills*. Basingstoke: Palgrave.

Eaton, N. and Moule, P. (2006) Assessment and evaluation. In: Glenn, S. and Moule, P. (eds) *E-learning in Nursing*. Basingstoke: Palgrave.

Eysenbach, G. and Till, J.E. (2001) Ethical issues in qualitative research on Internet communities. *British Medical Journal* 323: 1103–1105.

Maier, P. and Warren, A. (2000) *Integrating Technology in Learning and Teaching: A Practical Guide for Educators*. London: Kogan Page.

Moloney, M.F., Dietrich, A.S., Strickland, O. and Myerburg, S. (2003) Using Internet discussion boards as virtual focus groups. *Advances in Nursing Science* 26 (4): 274–286.

Morgan, C. and O'Reilly, M. (1999) *Assessing Open and Distance Learners*. London: Kogan Page.

Simpson, O. (2002) *Supporting Students in Online, Open and Distance Learning*. London: Kogan Page.

Recommended further reading

Cottrell, S. (2003) *The Study Skills Handbook*. Basingstoke: Palgrave Macmillan.

Appendix: Alphabetical list of websites and URLs used in this book

Adobe Acrobat Reader: this is free software that can be downloaded free of charge http://www.adobe.com/products/acrobat/readstep2.html
AltaVista http://www.altavista.com
Ask.com (Teoma) http://www.ask.com
BBC 'My Web My Way' http://www.bbc.co.uk/accessibility/
British Library http://www.bl.uk
Child Welfare Information Gateway http://www.childwelfare.gov
Cochrane Library http://www.thecochranelibrary.com
ComScore http://www.comscore.com/press/release.asp?press=849
Depression and Bi-polar Support Alliance http://www.dbsalliance.org/Info/supportgroups.html#
Download.com http://www.download.com
E-Learning Research Centre http://www.elrc.ac.uk
EndNote (referencing manager) http://www.endnote.com
European Computer Driving Licence (ECDL) http://www.ecdl.com
Excite http://www.excite.com
Google http://www.google.co.uk or http://www.google.com (Google.co.uk – and versions from other countries such as www.google.com.au for Australia etc. – gives you the opportunity to search just within web pages from the United Kingdom)
Health On the Net (HON) http://www.hon.ch
HotBot http://www.hotbot.com
InfoVoyager at the University of Hull http://www.infovoyager.hull.ac.uk/index2.html
Intute http://www.intute.ac.uk
Lycos mail http://mail.lycos.com
Medical Matrix http://medmatrix.org
MSN Hotmail (email) http://join.msn.com/hotmail/
MSN Messenger http://messenger.msn.com
National Library for Health http://www.library.nhs.uk
New Molton virtual online town http://www.wlv.ac.uk/molt
Penfield Virtual Hospital http://www.hud.ac.uk/hhs/departments/nursing/penfield_site

PowerPoint Reader http://www.microsoft.com/downloads
ProCite (referencing manager) http://www.procite.com
Quick Time Player http://www.apple.com/quicktime/win.html
Real Player http://uk.real.com/
Reference Manager http://www.refman.com
Ripfa: Research in Practice for Adults http://www.ripfa.org.uk
Royal College of Nursing http://www.rcn.org.uk
Social Care online http://www.scie-socialcareonline.org.uk
Study Skills http://www.palgrave.com/skills4study/
Thames Valley Police Chat Safe
    http://www.thamesvalley.police.uk/chatsafe/young.htm
Wannadoo (email) http://www.wanadoo.co.uk/communicate/email/
Windows Media Player http://www.microsoft.com/windows/windows
    media
Yahoo! Messenger http://messenger.yahoo.com
Yahoo! Mail http://mail.yahoo.com/
Yahoo! Search http://search.yahoo.com

Glossary

Technical terms and abbreviations are highlighted in bold in the text. The following list explains the meaning of these terms.

Advanced search   A facility in Internet and electronic database search engines that allows more complex searching using more than one term and the ability to search for specific types of entry such as author names and journal titles.

Archive   A repository that holds files and documents that are no longer required regularly by users, but may be required later. The files are stored out of the main view, but can be accessed easily if needed.

Attachments   This refers to files that can be 'attached' to an email message in their original format. It allows things like word processed files and photographs to be sent to the receiver, who can download directly to their own computer from the email message.

Back-up   The process of making extra copies of files to be stored in a different place or medium from the original. This is an essential safety process. Computer files and the materials on which they are stored can easily be damaged or corrupted and become unusable. Back-up files make sure that other copies of your work can be accessed if problems occur.

Blended learning   A mixture of learning and teaching modes that includes traditional classroom and tutorial methods as well as some of the online and electronic methods discussed in this book. This is a common approach in health and social care.

Boolean operators   Boolean logic is a simple system for allowing you to combine terms for an electronic search, so that you are asking the search engine to look for specific combinations of words. These are useful in all kinds of search engines to enable you to be more specific about what you are looking for and identify materials that are more specific to your needs, thus narrowing your searches down and helping to avoid less appropriate material. The three main 'operators' or terms in the system are: AND, OR, AND NOT.

Broadband   A way of transmitting large amounts of data, voice and video via the Internet at a greater speed and higher quality than through normal telephone networks. A broadband Internet connection is advisable for e-learning students as it enables them to access media like video files from the Internet more easily.

CD – see **Compact disc**

Chat/chat room   A chat room is a virtual room. It is a computer window that you use to communicate with others in real time. You type messages and they appear on the computer screens of the people who are in the room at the same time. This is known as synchronous chat, in that it happens simultaneously.

Communities of practice   An online community of practice is a group of professional practitioners, often from the same or related professional background, who come together to share ideas and experiences, to learn and to tackle professional and work-based problems and issues.

Compact Disc/CD/CD-Rom   CDs are compact discs that are used for permanently or temporarily storing computer data or files. They look similar to CDs used in the music industry. CDs quite often need a special software package to allow you to save (or 'burn') data onto them and some are 'non-rewritable' in that once data is stored on them it can't be wiped and replaced. 'Rom' stands for read only memory. This means that the data can only be accessed, but not altered, by the user.

Constructivism   A theory of learning and teaching that argues that students construct their own knowledge. It sees learning as a dynamic process in which the learner constructs new ideas or concepts on their current or past knowledge and in response to the learning situation they are in. Constructivism implies that learners do not passively absorb information but construct it themselves and that the teacher is a facilitator of this.

Copy and paste   A common facility in many computer systems that allows you to copy chunks of material from one document and place it in another while leaving the previous document exactly as it is.

Corrupted/corruption   A change in computer data such that the data content received is not what was originally sent and is often unusable.

Crash/crashed   Computers can be temperamental. This term means that the computer has a 'frozen' screen or is not functioning properly in some way. Most people tend to switch off their computer and restart it, sometimes known as rebooting.

Cyberplace/cyberspace   The virtual (nebulous or unreal) 'place' where humans interact over computer networks. Describes the world of connected computers and the society that gathers around them. To many people the Internet does feel like a real place where their lives are conducted on a day-to-day basis.

Data   A wide variety of types of information stored on a computer system and used to accomplish computer tasks. Often this is factual information contained in text or numerical format. Your computer converts this information into a digital format for storage and processing.

Database   A computer package that allows the storage, sorting and searching of large amounts of complex data or information.

Dial-up   An older way of connecting to the Internet using a normal telephone line. This is the precursor of broadband Internet access and is becoming less common.

Digital   Information recorded electronically using a method of storing, processing and transmitting information through the use of distinct electronic or optical pulses that represent the binary digits 0 and 1. Most electronic media is referred to as digital. In this book we refer to images, audio files and video material, for example, created in this way as digital.

Discs/disks   A physical place or piece of computer equipment where data can be stored. There are a number of different portable forms of data storage such as floppy disks, CDs and flash drives, for example.

Discussion board   A communication tool used commonly in e-learning and online communities. It is asynchronous in that you do not need to be logged on at the same time as other users. Messages can be left and group members can log on and off at any time to read and reply to messages. Conversations or discussions take place over a period of time.

Download/downloadable   The process of taking materials and files from the Internet and saving them to your own computer.

Drop box   A kind of electronic 'mail box' where you can post work such as essays for your tutor or other students to collect. It is almost like an online sorting office.

Dropdown menu   A way of accessing different features of a computer system such as a word processing package. A menu whose title is normally visible but whose contents are shown only when the user clicks on the title or a small arrow next to the title The menu items then appear below the title. The user may select an item from the menu by dragging the mouse from the menu title to the item and releasing, or by clicking the title and then clicking the item.

E-books   Books published online – they look exactly the same as the print version, but you can download them from the Internet. Many universities offer a growing number of e-books via their online catalogue.

E-journals   Journals and periodicals that are published online. They are often identical to the print version. They can usually be accessed via your university or college library web pages. You can also subscribe to them individually. Some are published on the Internet only – others also have print versions. Some of them have free access on the Internet.

E-learning   The online delivery of education and training using a variety of electronic systems and methods.

Electronic database/electronic resource   An electronically searchable source of information usually available on the Internet. In health and social care these usually facilitate a search for literature or information on a given subject.

Email   An electronic means of sending typed text similar to a letter or message from one computer to another using an Internet connection. This mail is almost instantaneously delivered to the recipient. Email is becoming a widespread feature of everyday life at work and at home.

Emoticons   One way to include emotional expression in your message postings. These are typed characters that often use keyboard characters to give the impression of a facial expression, to indicate an emotion or attitude, for example to indicate intended humour. There are also some abbreviations used to express emotions, which are also commonly used in mobile telephone text messaging.

E-tivities   Online activities usually created by an e-learning tutor for the purposes of facilitating student learning.

European Computer Driving Licence (ECDL)   A widely recognized qualification across Europe that demonstrates the holder's competence in basic computer skills.

Extranet   The part of a company or organization's internal computer network, which is available to outside users, for example, information services for customers.

Face-to-face   A term often used to denote forms of communication that involve the actual meeting of two or more individuals. In e-learning the term is used as the opposite to online communication.

Favourites   A list of your favourite, essential or most used websites held by your computer's web browser to make it easier for you to access sites that you use often.

Flash drive/USB flash drive   A small, lightweight, removable data storage device. These are portable mass data storage devices, which means that they can store large amounts of data. They are often known as 'memory sticks'. They are little pieces of equipment that can be purchased with various memory capacities. Their main advantage is that they allow the storage of larger computer files than CDs and floppy disks and they are very small, making portability easy. They come with their own piece of embedded software for organizing the files and connect easily into one of the ports (or holes) known as the USB port, which is specifically designed for plugging in external devices to a computer.

Floppy disk   The smallest kind of data storage that tends to operate from the A: Drive in your computer.

Focus group   A group of individuals brought together, often for research purposes, to discuss an issue of interest. Focus groups are usually led by a facilitator and focus on a specific issue or area of interest. They are also used in market research and policy development.

Formative assessment   Assessment processes that are used to support learning. They are not formally assessed but the student is given feedback to help them to see how they are progressing.

Gateways/portals   Websites that provide access to lots of other websites and materials. The links to other sites are often assessed for their suitability by the people who run the gateway or portal.

Globalization/globalized A term used to denote the way in which the world has become a smaller place and enables us to think in terms of worldwide issues rather than just local ones. The advent of cheap travel and the Internet are seen as major catalysts for this.

Hand search The process of looking at the indexes or contents lists of journals to ascertain if material of use is present when searching for literature on a certain subject. This often produces more accurate results than database searches.

Hard copies Paper printed versions of materials also found in electronic format.

Hard drive A large electronic data storage compartment in your computer – it is often also known as the C: Drive.

Hits Refers to the number of results when an Internet or database search is carried out.

Home page The front page of a website that acts as an access point for all other pages and contains the main menu for the site.

HTML/Hypertext Mark-up Language A term for the language that your computer uses to make material readable from and on the Internet. Files available in HTML do not need any specific software other than a web browser to open them and they take up less memory because they are in a simpler format.

Hyperlink A piece of text within an electronic file that, when clicked, takes the user to a specific site or page on the Internet or on their computer or network. The link is usually underlined or in a different text colour. It means that the user can swap quickly to another file that contains related information.

Inbox/outbox The mail boxes that contain your electronic mail. The inbox contains email that has been sent to you and the outbox contains email that you have sent to others.

Information and communications technology (ICT)/information technology (IT)/IC&T Generic terms that mean the whole of computer and telecommunications systems.

Internet A worldwide network of computers.

Internet browser – see **Web browser**

Internet café A place on the high street where you can access computers with an Internet connection. There is usually a charge for this service, which varies greatly but can be very reasonable away from the centre of main tourist destinations. Sometimes coffee is available and sometimes not!

Internet telephony The use of the Internet to make the equivalent of telephone calls using the spoken word at very low cost. Requires the use of a microphone connected to a computer.

Intranet An internal network of interconnected computers within a specific organization.

Junk mail – see **Spam**

Learning journal A log of reflections on the learning processes and experiences by an individual student.

Log in/log on/logging in/logging on   Refers to the process of entering a computer system, often requiring the use of specific user names and passwords.

Lurker/lurking   Reading messages in discussion forums and chat rooms without responding to the discussion in any way is known as lurking.

Managed Learning Environment   An Internet-based system used for learning. The system is used for sharing of learning materials and online communication. Managed environments also contain systems for keeping track of students' details and progress.

Memory stick – see **Flash drive**

Multimedia   The use of different kinds of media such as images, audio, video and text as well as computer generated animation. Computer generated animation is also used extensively in the creation of animated films for the film industry.

Netiquette   Taken from the word etiquette, this covers the rules that apply to online communication. It is a code of conduct that means you should be polite when working in online discussions and chats and avoid saying and doing things that might upset others.

Network/networked   A network is a computer connection that allows a number of people to access the information available on that computer system at the same time, but spread over a larger geographical area. Networked information and facilities are available via a computer connection (usually the Internet) accessible to more than one person at the same time.

New thread – see **Thread**

Online   When you are connected to the Internet, you are said to be online.

Outbox – see **Inbox**

Password/user name   A combination of letters and/or numbers that are specific to you. These are used to access computers and computer systems such as websites and virtual learning environments to protect them from use by people who are not authorized to use them.

Paste – see **Copy and paste**

Pod cast   A method where sound or video files, broadcast on the radio for example, can be downloaded by a user. Users can subscribe, often free, to pod casts that are automatically downloaded to their computer as soon as they are available. The user can then download them to a portable device such as an MP3 Music or DVD player.

Pop-up   Small box of information that appears on your computer screen while you are looking at a website. Pop-ups are often used for advertising, but can also be used for chat rooms etc. They allow you to carry on working in a website while you have the additional source of information or activity at the same time. They can also be a nuisance.

Pop-up blocker   A system that prevents pop-ups from appearing on your computer screen.

Portable Document Format file/PDF file   A file that is created in such a way that it can be viewed but not altered by another user.

Portals – see **Gateways**

Post/posting   A term that refers to the messages that you leave in a discussion board or forum.

PowerPoint®   One of Microsoft's suite of computer packages. PowerPoint® is used by tutors and others to make lively presentations for teaching.

Rebooting   Restarting a computer.

Search engine   A tool for searching for specific information within a website or database.

Simulated learning   The use of contrived situations that are designed to be as close to the real world as possible but enable students to practise skills in a relatively safe environment. In health care dummies or manikins are often used for this and in social care role play it is a common option. Such simulations can also be delivered online.

Software/software package   A computer program, package or system that can be loaded onto your computer to provide a specific facility.

Spam/junk mail   This is the unsolicited, unwanted, irrelevant or inappropriate sending of emails in mass quantities, commonly as an advertising ploy.

Spell-checker   A useful facility in lots of computer systems that allows you to click on a button and check all the spelling in the document or text you have created. Spelling mistakes are highlighted and you are given the opportunity to choose the correct word or spelling from a suggested list. Some systems offer grammar checks in a similar way.

Spreadsheet   A computer program that uses tables to organize numerical data and provides analysis of the date.

Streaming – see **Video streaming**

Sub-menu   A menu that appears when an item in a previous menu is clicked in order to offer a series of further options.

Summative assessment   Assessment in a course or module, the results of which contribute to the final mark or judgement of that module.

Surfing   The process of exploring the Internet.

Synchronous chat – see **Chat**

Text language   Shortened forms of words that are used to reduce the numbers of characters in a mobile phone text message or chat room message.

Thread/new thread   A specific topic of conversation within an online discussion board or forum. New threads are created when the topic changes.

Tools menu   A drop-down menu in a computer program that allows the user to conduct a number of tasks within the programme.

URL/Uniform Resource Locator   This is the address of a page on the Internet that often (but not always) begins http:// or www.

USB flash drive – see **Flash drive**

User name – see **Password**

Video conferencing   A system that enables two or more people to use a telephone line or computer system to view moving and talking pictures of each other and conduct conversations without being physically near each other.

Video streaming   Playing a video as it is downloaded from the Internet so that it begins to play as soon as the first part is available and while the remainder is still downloading. This means that the file does not need to be stored on the computer in the first instance. The video file is decompressed so that it plays much more quickly and reliably.

Virtual learning environment/VLE   A system that enables students to access learning materials online and a series of communication tools for working with their e-learning tutors and other students.

Web/World Wide Web/WWW   The network, also known as the Internet, that enables millions of computers to be connected together.

Web browser/Internet browser   A computer program that enables access to and exploration of the Internet.

Web page   Each page within a website is known as a web page and it has its own address.

Website   A site or location on the Internet or World Wide Web. Each website usually contains a home page, which is the first document users see when they enter the site. The site might also contain additional pages. Each site is owned and managed by an individual, company, or organization.

Wireless/wireless network   A radio wave system that is used to enable users to connect to the Internet without the need for a wire connected to a telephone line.

Word processing/word processor   The creation, input, editing and production of words in documents and texts by use of a specific computer system.

World Wide Web – see **Web**

Index